The Premenstrual Syndromes

CONTEMPORARY ISSUES IN OBSTETRICS AND GYNECOLOGY

VOLUME 2

SERIES EDITORS

Nathan G. Kase, M.D.
Richard L. Berkowitz, M.D.

Volumes Already Published

Forthcoming Volumes in the Series

THE PREMENSTRUAL SYNDROMES

Guest Editor

Leslie Hartley Gise, M.D.

Associate Clinical Professor and Associate Director
Liaison Division, Department of Psychiatry
Director, Premenstrual Syndromes Program and Liaison Psychiatrist
Department of Obstetrics–Gynecology and Reproductive Science
Mount Sinai School of Medicine of the City University of New York
New York, New York

Series Editors

Nathan G. Kase, M.D.

Dean
Mount Sinai School of Medicine of the City University of New York
New York, New York

Richard L. Berkowitz, M.D.

Professor and Chairman,
Department of Obstetrics–Gynecology and Reproductive Science
Mount Sinai School of Medicine of the City University of New York
New York, New York

CHURCHILL LIVINGSTONE
New York, Edinburgh, London, Melbourne
1988

Library of Congress Cataloging in Publication Data

The Premenstrual syndromes.

(Contemporary issues in obstetrics and gynecology;
v. 2)
    Includes bibliographies and index.
    1. Premenstrual syndrome. I. Gise, Leslie Hartley.
II. Series. [DNLM: 1. Premenstrual Syndrome.
W1 CO769MRH v.2 / WP 560 P925]
RG165.P745   1988   618.1'72   87-26814
ISBN 0-443-08537-4

© **Churchill Livingstone Inc. 1988**

Distributed in the United Kingdom by Churchill
Livingstone, Robert Stevenson House, 1-3 Baxter's Place,
Leith Walk, Edinburgh EH1 3AF, and by associated
companies, branches, and representatives throughout the
world.

Accurate indications, adverse reactions, and dosage
schedules for drugs are provided in this book, but it is
possible that they may change. The reader is urged to review
the package information data of the manufacturers of the
medications mentioned.

Acquisitions Editor: *Linda Panzarella*
Copy Editor: *Ann Ruzycka*
Production Designer: *Jill Little*
Production Supervisor: *Jane Grochowski*

Printed in the United States of America

First published in 1988

To Tom, Robin, and my mother
for their love and support

CONTRIBUTORS

Sheryle W. Alagna, Ph.D. Associate Professor, Department of Medical Psychology, Uniformed Services University of the Health Sciences, F. Edward Hébert School of Medicine, Bethesda, Maryland; Research Associate, Institute for Research on Women's Health, Inc., Washington, D.C.

James B. Brown, Ph.D., D.C.S. Professor, Department of Obstetrics and Gynaecology, University of Melbourne, Royal Women's Hospital, Melbourne, Victoria, Australia

Graham D. Burrows, M.D., Ch.B., B.Sc., D.P.M., F.R.A.N.Z.C.P., F.R.C. Psych. Professor and Director, Department of Psychiatry, University of Melbourne, Austin Hospital and Larundel Hospital, Heidelberg, Victoria, Australia

Virginia Cassara, M.A., M.S.S.W. Executive Director, PMS Action, Irvine, California

C. James Chuong, M.D. Assistant Professor, Division of Reproductive Endocrinology and Infertility, and Director, Premenstrual Syndrome Clinic, Department of Obstetrics and Gynecology, University of Texas Medical Branch at Galveston, Galveston, Texas

Carolyn B. Coulam, M.D. Medical Director, Methodist Center for Reproduction and Transplantation Immunology, Methodist Hospital of Indiana, Inc., Indianapolis, Indiana

Lorraine Dennerstein, M.B., B.S., Ph.D., D.P.M., F.R.A.N.Z.C.P. First Assistant and President, International Society of Psychosomatic Obstetrics and Gynaecology, and Founder and Past-President, Australian Society of Psychosomatic Obstetrics and Gynaecology, Department of Psychiatry, The University of Melbourne, Heidelberg, Victoria, Australia

Jean Endicott, Ph.D. Professor of Clinical Psychology, Department of Psychiatry, Columbia University College of Physicians and Surgeons; Chief, Research Assessment and Training Department, New York State Psychiatric Institute, New York, New York

Elizabeth Farrell, M.B.B.S., M.R.C.O.G., F.R.A.C.O.G. Consultant Gynaecologist, Menstrual and Menopause Clinic, Monash Medical Centre, Clayton, Victoria; Assistant Gynaecologist, Royal Melbourne Hospital, Carlton, Victoria, Australia

Ellen Freeman, Ph.D. Research Associate Professor, Departments of Obstetrics and Gynecology and Psychiatry, University of Pennsylvania School of Medicine, Philadelphia, Pennsylvania

Sharon Golub, Ph.D. Professor, Department of Psychology, College of New Rochelle, New Rochelle, New York; Adjunct Professor, Department of Psychiatry, New York Medical College, Valhalla, New York

Gordon Gotts, B.Sc., M.Sc. Psychologist and Lecturer, Swinburne College of Tafe, Hawthorn, Victoria, Australia

Uriel Halbreich, M.D. Professor and Director of Biobehavioral Research, Department of Psychiatry, State University of New York at Buffalo School of Medicine, Buffalo, New York

Jean A. Hamilton, M.D. Research Associate, Department of Behavioral Sciences, University of Chicago; Research Associate, Department of Psychiatry, Michael Reese Medical Center, Chicago, Illinois; Scientific Director, Institute for Research on Women's Health, Inc., Washington, D.C.

Elizabeth Holtzman, J.D. District Attorney, King's County, Brooklyn, New York

William Henry Keppel, M.D. Staff Psychiatrist, Emile Gamelin Institute, Portland, Oregon

Wayne S. Maxson, M.D. Director, Northwest Center for Infertility and Reproductive Endocrinology, Margate, Florida

Bruce S. McEwen, Ph.D. Professor and Head, Laboratory of Neuroendocrinology, The Rockefeller University, New York, New York

Carol Morse, M.Ed.Psych., M.A.P.S.S. Research Fellow, Department of Psychiatry, University of Melbourne, Austin Hospital, Heidelberg, Victoria; Consulting Psychologist, Menstrual–Menopause Disorders Clinic, Monash Medical Centre, Clayton, Victoria, Australia

Howard J. Osofsky, M.D., Ph.D. Professor and Head, Department of Psychiatry, Louisiana State University School of Medicine; Teaching Analyst, New Orleans Psychoanalytic Institute, New Orleans, Louisiana

Barbara L. Parry, M.D. Assistant Professor, Department of Psychiatry, University of California, San Diego, School of Medicine, La Jolla, California

Jeffrey L. Rausch, M.D. Assistant Professor, Department of Psychiatry, University of California, San Diego, School of Medicine, La Jolla, California

Karl Rickels, M.D. Professor of Psychiatry and Stuart and Emily B.H. Mudd Professor of Human Behavior, University of Pennsylvania School of Medicine, Philadelphia, Pennsylvania

Margery A. Smith, Ph.D. Senior Lecturer, Department of Obstetrics and Gynaecology, University of Melbourne, Royal Women's Hospital, Melbourne, Victoria, Australia

Steven J. Sondheimer, M.D. Associate Professor, Department of Obstetrics and Gynecology, University of Pennsylvania School of Medicine, Philadelphia, Pennsylvania

PREFACE

Premenstrual syndrome (PMS) is a controversial condition affecting both mind and body. Widely varying symptoms and uncoordinated efforts in research have made it difficult to profile this complex disorder. Because of its psychobiological nature, no one discipline has taken responsibility for treatment. Women continue to seek help while the medical professions debate whether to treat PMS as a fad or an ailment.

PMS does exist. In fact, there are probably many syndromes. Although *PMS* is used for convenience, *premenstrual changes* is a more accurate term. It implies that these changes are diversified and should be studied as subtypes of a disease rather than as a specific syndrome.

It is in this setting that this book was conceived. Our purpose is to bring together in one volume the topics in which current research is being done relative to PMS. It is hoped that this material will help physicians and other health professionals evaluate and treat patients, critically evaluate the literature, plan research, and educate the public in a responsible and informed fashion.

To accomplish this goal, 25 contributors representing a wide spectrum of interests have written chapters that address the problems of patient history, evaluation, diagnosis and treatment, and report the latest findings in psychology, neuroendocrinology, nutrition, and pharmacology. This book is at the same time scientific, with reports of basic research, and clinical, with helpful information for the primary care physicians who diagnose and treat the PMS patient. It is intended to emphasize the information that is currently available as well as to present the controversies surrounding PMS. Further, it informs the practitioner of the broad spectrum of scholarly, legal, and social concern for and interest in premenstrual changes.

Premenstrual changes cannot be viewed as some skeptical cynics have proclaimed as yet another diversion of the "worried well," absorbing time and energy to no avail. There is something important going on here, quite possibly a portal to understanding much of human behavioral variability and reactivity. It deserves unimpassioned critical review. We hope our readers agree.

I give special thanks to Dr. Nathan Kase for his full support of the conference and this volume. Thanks also to Minerva Brown, Director, The Page and William Black Post Graduate School, Mount Sinai Medical Center, and to the Upjohn Company and the Ortho Pharmaceutical Corporation for their help.

Leslie Hartley Gise, M.D.

CONTENTS

INTRODUCTION

The study of the premenstrual syndromes has omitted descriptive knowledge of premenstrual changes, including the natural history of these phenomena. Furthermore, the present knowledge of the premenstrual syndromes is limited by methodologic flaws in most of the research done to date.[1,2] PMS is not a single discrete entity or a specific syndrome, but a heterogeneous group of symptoms better named *premenstrual changes*.* This is more than a semantic difference. It implies that premenstrual changes should be studied as diversified subtypes. Why is it that all women do not have it? Why are the symptoms so variable? As a consequence of this heterogeneity, there is no universally accepted definition of PMS. Misinformed public opinion is another problem. Finally, the variable nature of this problem makes diagnosis difficult and to date, no medication has proven effective in alleviating the symptoms. Until these syndromes are better understood, efforts in classification and treatment may be misguided.

DEFINITION AND CLASSIFICATION

Premenstrual changes can be defined as "the cyclic occurrence of symptoms that are of sufficient severity to interfere with some aspects of life and which appear with consistent and predictable relationship to menses."[1] The National Institute of Mental Health (NIMH), in its Workshop on Premenstrual Syndrome (co-sponsored by the Center for Studies of Affective Disorders and the Psychobiological Processes and Behavioral Medicine Section), made an effort to delineate PMS from other disorders with two criteria: (1) A marked increase (about 30 percent) in the intensity of symptoms measured intermenstrually (from days 5 through 10 follicular), as compared to those measured premenstrually (within 6 days prior to menstruation), and (2) documentation of these changes for at least two consecutive cycles.[1]

In trying to define and classify the premenstrual syndromes, one must consider the fact that there are normal as well as pathological changes, and that up to 15 percent of women actually feel better prior to menstruation. This is a spectrum of changes from normal (affecting up to 95 percent of women) to pathological and incapacitating (affecting about 5 percent of women).

The inclusion of late luteal phase dysphoric disorder (LLDD) in the Appendix of the revised Diagnostic and Statistical Manual of the American

---

*Nevertheless, the term *PMS* is used in this volume for convenience.

Psychiatric Association (DSM-III-R)[2] is an encouraging sign in our effort to standardize definition and classification. The most important feature of this entry is the specification of 2 months of daily prospective recordkeeping to confirm diagnosis. However, the criteria for diagnosis are vague. On the one hand, the degree to which symptoms must change from one time of the month to the other is *not* specified, and on the other, the criterion that symptoms must remit "within a few days" after the onset of menses *is* specified. Traditionally, symptoms do remit within one to two days after the onset of menstruation, but some women state that symptoms persist for up to a week after menstruation starts, and the controversy as to whether these patterns should be identified as premenstrual changes is understandable.

Although the DSM-III-R states that symptoms are not to be "merely an exacerbation of . . . another disorder," it gives no way to determine whether mood swings, irritability, anxiety, or depression are caused by LLDD or by another disorder. Furthermore, it allows a provisional diagnosis to be made prior to confirmation by prospective ratings although there is substantial evidence that most women (about 80 percent) who report premenstrual changes do not have their symptoms confirmed. Finally, recordkeeping for a period of 2 months is probably inadequate to diagnose a premenstrual syndrome because symptoms sometimes vary from month to month. It may take up to 12 months to confirm the existence of a premenstrual syndrome.

Should late luteal phase dysphoric disorder (LLDD) be classified as a psychiatric diagnosis? Because the relation of menstrual cycle to symptoms has been shown to be correlated but not causal, there is no scientific evidence to make LLDD a mental disorder. Postpartum depression and menopausal depression are not classified as psychiatric disorders, and no other psychiatric disorder has as many physical symptoms as LLDD. *Premenstrual tension* already is included in the International Classification of Diseases, 9th Revision, Clinical Modification (ICD-9-CM), which is coded on Axis III.[3] Premenstrual changes, then, can be coded on Axes I and III of the DSM-III-R. While this is confusing, it can be said that the reasons for classifying LLDD as a psychiatric diagnosis are practical, not scientific, and the manner of classification will not add to our knowledge.

At present, the natural history of the premenstrual syndromes is not known; nor has this group of heterogeneous disorders been divided into meaningful subgroups which can help predict outcome. In the face of large numbers of women flocking to use unproven and potentially harmful drugs, accurate descriptive study of these changes over time is critical while other research efforts continue to clarify the nature of these symptoms. Few women are truly incapacitated by PMS, and the vast majority have mild symptoms which can be helped without medication. For this reason, medical intervention is premature until naturalistic, descriptive, and nonintrusive study leads us to a better understanding of these problems.

ETIOLOGY

The causes of PMS are not only hormonal changes and stress, but a multitude of causes like many other illnesses. Weiner[4] discusses the heterogeneity of the traditional psychosomatic diseases, such as asthma and hypertension, each subtype with its own etiology, epidemiology, and pathophysiology. It is appropropriate in this context to consider his classification of causes of such illnesses as predisposing, precipitating, and sustaining. For hypertension, for example, there may be a genetic predisposing cause, a stress-related precipitating cause, and a dietary sustaining cause, e.g., eating salt.

For premenstrual syndromes, predisposing causes may include a past history or family history of mental illness or alcoholism, or a past history of sexual abuse. Precipitating causes may include the discontinuence of birth control pills, bilateral tubal ligation, or hysterectomy. Sustaining causes may be related to life-style issues such as diet (caffeine, sugar, alcohol), use of nicotine, exercise, or stress. Thus, like many other illnesses, the etiology of premenstrual changes is multidetermined. The implications of this heterogeneity have not been sufficiently appreciated. For example, treatment studies, especially drug studies, may be premature if different premenstrual syndromes are grouped together, and thereby are masking a treatment effect.

The observation of behavioral changes in baboons premenstrually suggests that there *are* hormonal determinants. But there are also social and psychological determinants. In women, premenstrual syndromes have at least 150 different symptoms that involve every specialty of medicine.

Because premenstrual changes affect both mind and body, many etiologies have been proposed. In addition to progesterone, for example, beta-endorphins, thyroid homones, and melatonin have been suspected causes. Since sex hormones affect neurotransmitters, hormonal changes may predispose to depression, which in turn may be triggered by either endocrine or environmental events. But no "one-substance" cause is likely to emerge. Most research has stressed biology and excluded psychology. Little psychological work has been done since 1939, when Benedek and Rubinstein predicted cycle phase from blindly rated transcriptions of psychoanalytic sessions and found women to be concerned with passivity and maternalism during the luteal phase.

Another conceptual issue is the challenge to develop a psychobiology of human experience in which premenstrual changes are viewed within the broader context of cyclic changes in mood and behavior in both men and women.[5] Premenstrual changes have been singled out as a unique phenomenon. In reality, they are only one of a number of cyclic changes in mood and behavior observed in both men and women. This approach considers that the brains of male rats have estrogen receptors and that in certain parts of the brain testosterone is converted to estradiol. This approach looks at other cyclic changes such as "jet lag" or "Monday morning blues" shared by both men and women. One must ask how these cyclic changes compare to premenstrual changes. Furthermore, mood and behavior changes linked in time with reproduction are not necessarily unique to women even though the specific biologic changes are. For example, both men and women show mood changes linked to infertility despite the location of the biological problem in one or the other.

Although frequently associated with premenstrual changes, dysmenorrhea must be differentiated from them. Dysmenorrhea is associated with ovulatory cycles more than PMS, is unrelated to age (PMS usually gets worse with age), improves after childbirth (PMS usually does not), is basically a pain syndrome (pelvic pain is seldom a feature of PMS), and occurs *during* as opposed to *prior to* menstruation. The pathophysiology of dysmenorrhea is known, and the clinical response to prostaglandin synthetase inhibitors is clear.

The relationship of PMS to somatization is unclear. In some ways PMS patients resemble hypochondriacal patients who complain about physical symptoms and refuse to talk about feelings. Although PMS patients often present with the conviction that their hormones are at fault, it is typically easier for them to shift their focus to psychological and behavioral factors which may be aggravating their condition.

The relationship of PMS to psychotherapy is also unclear. Many PMS patients have had psychotherapy in the past. Does PMS serve to ward off further psychotherapy or to function as a resistance? These issues at the interface of gynecology and psychiatry need more study.

ATTITUDES

There are negative attitudes toward menstruation in our culture. Indeed, sexist attitudes have contributed to the relative neglect of women's health issues. Like many problems in psychobiology, PMS falls through the cracks, and no one discipline wants to take responsibility for it. Gynecologists send PMS patients to psychiatrists and psychiatrists send them to gynecologists.

Many people think of menstruation as a disease where the menstruating woman is disabled, or is suffering from some impairment. Because the menstrual cycle is a biological phenomenon associated with women, premenstrual changes even have become connected with sex-role identification and issues of gender quality. Despite the fact that no studies confirm women's complaints that they cannot think clearly before or during menstruation, millions of people in this country believe that a woman truly cannot function as well as usual while menstruating, and indeed, believe that menstruation affects a woman's ability to think. In light of this public opinion, feminists understandably have concern about the resultant accusations against women that they are "impaired" before or during menstruation, or that if they have PMS, they are a discredit to all women. Researchers, on the other hand, have examined the complexity of PMS, and have had the tendency to oversimplify the issues and have as a result limited the scope of their inquiries. They have tended to assume a biological cause and a specific drug cure, which has encouraged premature translation of basic research findings into treatment plans.

DETECTION AND REFERRAL

PMS represents a problem in detection and requires screening by primary care physicians. While PMS is overemphasized by some women, it is neglected by others who fail to tell their doctors about their symptoms for fear they are "going crazy." Since many women do not connect their symptoms to their menstrual cycle, they should be asked about premenstrual changes and premenstrual changes should be considered during the assessment of any intermittent or fluctuating symptoms in women of reproductive age. Premenstrual changes easily can be misdiagnosed as psychopathology, treatment failure, drug effect, or lack of pathology. All this depends on the time of the month a woman is seen, and her response to the physicians questions. Both physicians and public need further education to increase awareness and detection of menstrually related conditions.

Most major depression is not detected or treated and most depression occurs in women.[6] The life-cycle approach is crucial to understand reproductive-related depression in women. Women get depressed not only in association with the menstrual cycle, but also with menarche, use of oral contraceptives, pregnancy, infertility, perinatal loss, and menopause. Routinely asking women about psychological reactions associated with reproduction yields a clear history of major depressive episodes which would otherwise be undetected on routine medical or psychiatric examination.

Menstrual-cycle influences on various illnesses (allergies, migraine headaches, epilepsy, depression, and other psychiatric problems), drug metabolism (aspirin, insulin, antiepileptics, lithium and benzodiazepines), and physiology (oral glucose tolerance) do exist, but have largely been ignored. These influences may help explain the complexity and heterogeneity of syndromes observed by clinicians.

Drug and alcohol problems are commonly observed among women seeking treatment for premenstrual symptoms. Anecdotal reports of premenstrually increased drug and alcohol abuse have not yet been corroborated with systematic studies. The premenstrually increased abuse of drugs and alcohol among normal women as well as among women with diagnosed substance abuse is critical to understand women's mood and behavior changes. The suggestion that tolerance for alcohol is reduced premenstrually is an intriguing one which also deserves systematic study.

The chapters in this volume were originally presented as papers in "Premenstrual Syndrome: New Findings and Controversies," a symposium held at the Mount Sinai School of Medicine in New York City. They have been thoroughly updated and edited to comprise a book that is the only compilation to date of both gynecological and psychiatric perspective, as well as results of current research on the biochemistry and pharmacology of PMS. This material should help physicians and other health professionals assess and treat patients, critically evaluate the literature, plan research, and educate the public in a responsible and informed fashion.

Critical elements in future research will be good hypotheses, attention to methodology, including careful diagnosis and follow-up, as well as integration of biological and psychological variables. The search for quick answers and miracle drug cures does not solve the problem and does injustice to women suffering from these enigmatic disorders. A broad scope of awareness of the many aspects of the premenstrual syndromes should be the basis of new investigations into the etiology, epidemiology, and pathophysiology of the premenstrual syndromes.

REFERENCES

1. Endicott J, Halbreich U, Schacht S, Nee S: Premenstrual changes and affective disorders. Psychosom Med 43:519, 1981
2. Rubinow DR, Roy-Byrne P: Premenstrual syndromes: Overview from a methodologic perspective. Am J Psychiatry 141, 2:163, 1984
3. Workshop on Premenstrual Syndrome, co-sponsored by the Center for Studies of Affective Disorders and the Psychobiological Processes and Begavioral Medicine Section, Clinical Research Branch, National Institute on Mental Health, Rockville, MD, April 14–15, 1983
4. American Psychiatric Association: Diagnostic and Statistical Manual of Mental Disorders, Third Edition, Revised. American Psychiatric Association, Washington, DC, 1987
5. International Classification of Diseases, 9th Revision, Clinical Modification. 3 vols. Revisionist Press, Brooklyn, New York, 1984
6. Weiner, H: Psychobiology and Human Disease. Elsevier/North-Holland, New York, 1977
7. Hamilton JA: Psychobiology in context: Reproductive-related events in men's and women's lives. (Review of Brockington IF: Motherhood and Mental Illness, Grune & Stratton, New York, 1982.) Contemp Psychiatry 3, 1: 12 1984
8. Myers JK, Weissman MM, Tischler GL, et al: Six-month prevalence of psychiatric disorders in three communities: Arch Gen Psychiatry 41:959, 1984

1

Practical Problems in Evaluation

Jean Endicott
Uriel Halbreich

Many of us have had personal experience with premenstrual changes either in ourselves or in significant others. It is also true that syndromes that appear premenstrually are seen at other times, in men as well as in women. Possibly premenstrual changes can serve as a model to help us understand not only the pathophysiology of changes in mood and behavior during the menstrual cycle but also similar changes that appear at other times in women as well as in men.

This chapter summarizes some of the practical problems facing investigators and clinicians who focus on premenstrual changes. The findings reported here and the issues discussed have been covered in greater detail elsewhere.[1-7]

The problem of definitions arises first. The ones we have chosen for use in our studies are similar to those being used in much of the research and clinical work now going on elsewhere.

A feature is considered to be associated with the premenstrual period (and part of what we refer to as premenstrual changes) if it appears exclusively or changes substantially during the premenstrual period. If a woman is anxious most of the time and severely anxious premenstrually, we call the difference a *premenstrual change*. If someone is generally easygoing, not irritable, but becomes irritable premenstrually, we call it a premenstrual change. The feature does not exist in the same form or severity immediately prior to the premenstrual period, and it disappears or returns to its usual state or level of severity during menses. It is often said that these features switch back to their usual state at the start of menses, but careful data recording discloses that with most women it does not exactly switch: rather, it starts to recede, and by the end of menses generally it is gone or has returned to the usual level. As a result it is best to study women during their most stable period, or during the interval when there are the fewest problems, which is the week after menses.

1

The duration of premenstrual changes also varies considerably from one woman to the next. In some, daily ratings show that changes start around the time of ovulation and may remain noticeable for 10, 12, or even 14 days. The average length of premenstrual problems is around 5 days, so that women who seek treatment are usually having problems for about 7 to 10 days, including the few days after menses start.

METHODS OF EVALUATION

There are many ways of evaluating premenstrual changes. The most common, aside from a woman consulting the physician, social worker, or counselor to discuss premenstrual changes and problems, is the use of retrospective questionnaires. A woman is given a questionnaire with a number of items and asked to describe changes she has noticed: what her changes are like premenstrually and nonpremenstrually. On the questionnaire we developed women are asked to note the changes they believe are characteristic of their premenstrual period. Interviews are also used, sometimes just once during the premenstrual period. However, such an interview does not show the contrast between the premenstrual period and the postmenstrual or nonpremenstrual period. Generally we recommend that women be seen, if possible, during the premenstrual period and the week after menses.

Daily ratings by the subject are almost indispensable when evaluating the pattern of changes (i.e., their onset and offset) as well as determining which changes tend to be present each month (in contrast to changes that are present only alternate months or at other times). We assume that the changes result from an interaction between biologic vulnerability and life events; that is, when things are going fairly well, a subject may not display the kinds or severity of change during that cycle that might be present in another cycle when there is considerable stress.

Reports from significant others—spouses, siblings, roommates—are useful because a woman who is not particularly introspective may not be aware of some of the specific changes she displays or experiences. Such reports also help judge the severity of changes and the degree to which they impair social functioning, work, getting along with others, and other expected role behaviors.

When evaluating premenstrual changes, we find it valuable to look at the diversity of changes, not just at an overall "premenstrual syndrome." There should be enough specificity in the questionnaire item coverage to characterize changes in mood and behavior, as well as the physical changes, along the cycle. Generally we look at the entire cycle, because some women have momentary physical, mood, and behavioral changes around the time of ovulation that continue for a day or two. Sometimes they resemble a premenstrual change and sometimes they are quite different. It is thus important to know what the entire cycle is like, not just the premenstrual period. We try to obtain daily ratings on all the women in our studies throughout an entire cycle.

We are often asked, "What are the rates of premenstrual change?" The answer is, "It depends." It depends on what group of women are studied, how they are recruited, what their life stresses and history have been. For example, in the case of a depressive syndrome, i.e., a dysphoric mood with at least four associated symptoms (changes in sleep, appetite, energy level, concentration, thinking negative thoughts, feelings of guilt) but not necessarily social impairment, it becomes evident that 95 percent of women seeking treatment meet criteria for that category. Eighty-three percent of women in a depression clinic seeking treatment not for premenstrual changes but for chronic depression said they felt worse premenstrually. They noticed that, even though they were chronically depressed, the depression was worse during the premenstrual period. This observation is important in the treatment of chronically depressed or anxious women. In a sample group of student nurses (a class that filled out forms without having to sign them in exchange for a lecture), 51 percent said they noticed dysphoric changes in mood. On the other hand, a group of women executives who had "made it" in New York banks and law firms had the lowest rates of dysphoric changes. We have now studied about 14 defined groups, and the executives still have the lowest rates.

Regarding physical changes, various groups of women tend not to differ much during the menstrual cycle. Feelings of being bloated, of abdominal heaviness, of clothes not fitting well, and of rings and shoes feeling tight are found fairly consistently. Physical symptoms are relatively common, and there is little differentiation across groups of women, although women seeking treatment or who are chronically depressed tend to have somewhat more severe symptoms.

The problem that frequently causes women to seek treatment is hostility (the tendency to become irritable, have a low threshold for anger, be somewhat explosive) because it causes psychosocial difficulties with spouses, boyfriends, children, and co-workers. There is considerable differentiation across groups of women in regard to those who report hostile features on the questionnaire items, e.g., "I wake up feeling at war with the world," "I find myself more irritable," "I have a tendency to nag and complain," "I tend to fuss over small things," or physical violence: "I smash things like dishes, slam doors, break furniture." The latter is extremely rare, but feelings of irritability, hostility, and fussiness are not rare.

Hostile features were common in women who responded to television and newspaper announcements that we were studying premenstrual changes. Most women who came to a clinic for treatment of chronic depression also reported that they tend to be more irritable during the premenstrual period. On the other hand, student nurses and other medical center staff who responded to posted notices seeking subjects for studies during the menstrual cycle had relatively few hostile features.

Many clinicians and investigators do not realize that some women have bipolar changes premenstrually. There is a fortunate group—around 5 to 15 percent—who report having more energy, feeling better, getting more done, and being more creative. Some artists work better at this time. Other women report that they have a day or two when they feel more energetic—it may be a pleasant feeling, or it may have an unpleasant, driven quality—and then suddenly feel they do not want to do anything. One of our staff members who reported premenstrual fatigue wore an activity monitor for 2 months. After the first month, she said, "No wonder I'm tired! I didn't realize how much I did." Thinking that might have been an atypical month, she wore the monitor another month, and the contrast was even higher. She had 1 day of intense activity and then a day on which she felt like doing nothing.

There are several relatively common reasons for ruling out women from premenstrual treatment studies or other studies having to do with changes along the menstrual cycle. Most women seek treatment for self-diagnosed premenstrual changes or have been so diagnosed by their husband or physician. However, on daily ratings, some of these women are shown to have chronic depression or anxiety, and there may or may not be an increase premenstrually. We refer such women for treatment of the chronic depression or anxiety. There is another group of women with no clear-cut pattern, among whom the daily ratings show no stable relation to any phase of the menstrual cycle. Sometimes the patterns for these women are fairly flat, and sometimes they show changes with no set pattern. If the changes are severely disabling, we refer these women for treatment of their chronic difficulties. Clinicians who fail to obtain daily ratings for one or two full cycles risk studying or treating women who do not have clear-cut premenstrual changes.

In the past, when women complaining of premenstrual syndrome were treated with placebo, any improvement was attributed to the placebo. We have found that simply paying attention to the symptoms and making daily ratings tend to be therapeutic in several ways. For example, if a woman making daily ratings notices breast pain or a feeling of abdominal heaviness, she knows that it tends to precede the irritability and depression. She can then expect to be more sensitive during the next few days and perhaps warn family members to expect her impending mood, or she can try to reduce interactive problems temporarily. She is also much more conscious of having to watch her diet, alcohol intake, and some other actions that can make premenstrual symptoms worse. A woman who makes daily ratings for 1 month usually experiences a dampening down of the syndrome. If she is on any medication or placebo, she usually attributes the improvement to it. Therefore we ask each woman to record daily ratings for at least one cycle preceding treatment, as some women then find they do not need to take medication.

SCORING DAILY RATINGS

When we do have the daily ratings, how do we score them? First, as we are screening for the studies, we do an "eyeball" scoring. Certain clear-cut changes show up. A woman's chart may show that she becomes more and more irritable, reaching the highest score 2 days before the onset of menses and then gradually returning to her usual cheerful mood. Another woman may show she is quite irritable throughout the month, not every day perhaps but throughout the cycle, with no significant degree of change premenstrually. Rather than treating her for premenstrual syndrome, we would probably refer her for treatment of chronic problems.

The third pattern is one that shows nothing particularly associated with phases of the cycle. Changes may be going on throughout the month that are not related to the menstrual cycle at all. The fourth common pattern reveals ratings that show that not much is going on: The woman feels fine and has some premenstrual irritability, but not much.

It sounds as if the patterns of daily rating are easy to judge, but the reality is not so simple. For example, the pattern for a woman on whom we had 21 items across 41 days for two menstrual cycles raised a number of points. Some changes were consistent across both cycles, and some were not consistent. The middle period—after menses and prior to the luteal phase—tended to be "flat," but there are "blips" here and there that sometimes make scoring difficult. We also ask women to make notes on a "comment" page if anything happens that affected their physical condition or their mood. We then have some indication of how much reactivity there is, how much "noise", and can decide if these changes meet the criteria for our studies. In other words, there is no easy way to score daily ratings. One must review the report with the individual to determine what is really going on.

ASSOCIATION OF PREMENSTRUAL CHANGES WITH PSYCHOPATHOLOGY

Regarding the association of premenstrual syndromes with psychopathology, it must first be made clear that we do not consider premenstrual changes to be psychopathologic in themselves. Rather, they are phenomena that can reach the severity of a disorder if they cause significant impairment in work or social relations, or lead to suicide attempts, violence, or hospitalization. In other words, some women have behavioral changes that on a cross-sectional or longitudinal basis would be rated as indicating significantly impaired functioning.

Women who have a lifetime diagnosis of having had at least one period that met full RDC criteria or *DSM-III* criteria for a major depressive episode lasting at least 1 month are much more likely to have premenstrual depression than a similar group matched in age who have never had any kind of mental disorder, even minor affective syndromes or anxiety disorder, problems with alcohol or drugs, etc. There is usually not much difference in the water retention syndrome, but there is in the depressive syndrome. These results have been consistent across our series of studies as well as in studies done by other investigators. In women who have a lifetime diagnosis of major depressive disorder, premenstrual depression tends to run around 60 percent, with some studies finding it as high as 75 percent and others finding it somewhat lower, around 50 percent.

Likewise, there is evidence that a woman who has premenstrual depression is vulnerable to the development of a major depressive episode some time in her life. If she has had major depressive episodes in the past and has premenstrual dysphoria, she is probably more vulnerable to recurrences of the major depressive disorder.

Finally, when treating any mental or other medical disorder, the therapist should be alert to the phases of the patient's menstrual cycle. Many premenstrual symptoms are readily observable: headache, diarrhea, upset stomach, nausea, malaise, unusual fatigue, etc. Without such awareness, the symptoms may be attributed to side effects of medication or medication failure. One week to 10 days later, the new symptoms may disappear owing to phases of the menstrual cycle. Also, when treating chronic depression or anxiety, there may be a breakthrough of symptoms or a change in symptoms at the time of the premenstrual period. Both therapist and patient may tend to become discouraged, perhaps discontinuing therapy or trying other medications. However, if they know the woman is premenstrual, they can consider if there may be an alternative explanation for the negative changes.

At present there are no firm data on the etiology of premenstrual changes, and no treatment has been proved effective. It is highly unlikely that, given the great individual differences in women and the symptoms they manifest, a single etiology or therapeutic modality will be found. Only by focusing on the diversity of changes, trying different treatments for different subgroups of women, and conducting well controlled studies can we hope to discover effective treatment modalities or to isolate etiologic factors.

REFERENCES

1. Endicott J, Halbreich U, Schacht S, Nee J: Premenstrual changes and affective disorders. J Psychosomc Med 43:519, 1981
2. Halbreich U, Endicott J, Schacht S, Nee J: The diversity of premenstrual changes as reflected in the premenstrual assessment form. Acta Psychiatr Scand 65:46, 1982
3. Halbreich U, Endicott J, Nee J: Premenstrual depressive changes: value of differentiation. Arch Gen Psychiatry 40:535, 1983
4. Endicott J, Halbreich U: Retrospective report of premenstrual depressive changes: factors affecting confirmation by daily ratings. Psychopharmacol Bull 18:109, 1982
5. Harrison W, Sharpe L, Endicott J: Treatment of premenstrual syndrome. Gen Hosp Psychiatry 7:54, 1985
6. Halbreich U, Endicott J: Methodological studies of premenstrual changes. Psychoneuroendocrinology (in press)
7. Endicott J, Halbreich U, Schacht S, Nee J: Affective disorder and premenstrual depression. Syllabus, APA 137th Annual Meeting, Los Angeles, May 1984. APA Monographs (in press)

2

A Developmental Perspective

Sharon Golub

"Premenstrual Distress Gains Notice as a Chronic Issue in the Workplace," reads a January 22, 1986 *Wall Street Journal* headline. The article goes on to say that premenstrual syndrome (PMS) is a problem women try to hide, especially at work, for fear of reinforcing negative stereotypes about women. The myth of menstrual impairment persists despite almost 50 years of research that has shown no consistent demonstrable effect of the menstrual cycle on work or academic performance.

Professionals struggle with this double bind. The 1987 inclusion of late luteal phase dysphoric disorder (LLDD), a loosely defined variant of PMS, in the revised edition of the American Psychiatric Association's *Diagnostic and Statistical Manual of Mental Disorders* (*DSM-III-R*), has evoked a great deal of controversy. Some members of the American Psychiatric Association committee charged with revising the *DSM-III* believe that clarifying criteria for diagnosis will aid research and treatment; others, however, believe that the psychiatric label will stigmatize women as victims of their "raging hormones."

This controversy notwithstanding, perimenstrual symptoms are widespread. The most common symptoms are weight gain, headache, skin disorders, cramps, backache, fatigue, painful breasts, irritability, mood swings, anxiety, and depression. Studies differ as to the incidence of many of these symptoms, but several studies of United States and European non-clinical populations report a symptom incidence of more than 25 percent.[1-5] An international study conducted by the World Health Organization (WHO) in 10 countries in various parts of the world also found a high incidence of physical discomfort prior to or during menstruation (more than 50 percent), and 38 percent or more of the women sampled also indicated mood changes prior to or during menstruation.[6] Thus the data strongly suggest that a significant proportion of women are affected by menstrual symptoms. However, there is an important difference between incidence and degree. Many women experience mild to moderate symptoms, but only a relatively small number, about 2 to 8 percent, suffer disabling symptoms.[5]

The symptoms seem to divide fairly readily into two groups. Those symptoms more characteristic of the menstrual phase of the cycle are cramps, backache, tension, and fatigue. During the premenstruum symptoms such as irritability, depression, anxiety, water retention, and breast tenderness are more likely. Categorizing symptoms as menstrual or premenstrual is particularly useful when studying developmental changes, as the prevalence and intensity of each group appear to be age-related.

Thus symptoms of menstrual distress vary not only from woman to woman but also in the same woman at different times in her life. Anecdotal and research data suggest that young women more often experience dysmenorrhea and mood disturbances during menstruation, whereas older women are more likely to complain of premenstrual distress.[3,7-10] Premenstrual complaints have been reported to rise during the midtwenties and peak during the midthirties.[11-16]

When looking at the relation between age and menstrual symptoms, researchers are confronted with a number of methodologic problems. In addition to the usual ones, such as what are the measures and who are the subjects (normal women, gynecologic patients, school girls, prisoners, or some other select group), we must also ask about methods of birth control, parity, patterns of menstrual bleeding, and attitudes toward menstruation. Thus the complex interplay of physiologic, personality, experiential, and cultural variables must be addressed. There is a real need for longitudinal studies directed toward answering questions about menstrual cycle and menstrual symptom variability over the course of a woman's lifetime.

CULTURE AND ATTITUDES

It is difficult to ignore the pervasive negative mental set that exists regarding menstruation. We have only to look at some of the most popular terms used to allude to it: "the curse," "falling off the roof," "on the rag." Language shapes our perception of ourselves, and most menstrual expressions seem to be intended to maintain secrecy or avoid embarrassment. These attitudes are reinforced by the advertisements for sanitary products that seem to aim at making women anxious about "accidents" and present menstruation as messy, unpredictable, dirty, smelly, and, perhaps the biggest threat of all, something that can make one do "crazy things."

Menstrual blood has been considered both magical and poisonous, and the menstruating woman has often been seen as a danger to the community. Thus communities developed avoidance customs in order to protect themselves. In some cultures menstruating women were segregated and forbidden to cook for their husbands; and because menstrual blood was believed to be dangerous to men, sexual intercourse during menstruation was taboo.[17,18] Lest one think that these beliefs are long gone, see Table 2-1 for some of the beliefs and behaviors associated with menstruation found by WHO research-

A Developmental Perspective

TABLE 2-1.   **BELIEFS AND BEHAVIOR ASSOCIATED WITH MENSTRUATION:**
WHO STUDY

Belief/Behavior	Egypt (%)	Jamaica (%)	Korea (%)	Mexico (%)	Philippines (%)	UK (%)
Menstruation is necessary for femininity	96	61	79	57	95	42
Menstruation is dirty	88	33	34	53	41	7
Menstruation is like sickness	67	37	22	26	61	7
Intercourse should be avoided during menstruation	98	91	91	90	90	54
Visiting friends/relatives should be avoided during menstruation	55	39	7	16	24	0
Washing hair should be avoided during menstruation	16	21	11	14	68	5
Bathing should be avoided during menstruation	42	18	72	20	72	10

(Data from Snowden R, Christian B: Patterns and Perceptions of Menstruation. St. Martin's Press, New York, 1983.)

ers.[6] In Egypt 55 percent of the women believe that visits to friends and relatives should be avoided during menstruation. In many parts of the world, 90 percent or more of the people avoid intercourse during menstruation. Some of these menstrual injunctions exist in contemporary American culture as well. Perhaps the most common is the avoidance of sexual intercourse during menstruation; about half the population believes in abstaining. Do these people fear contamination or illness? Probably not. Many attribute their behavior to religious beliefs or aesthetic considerations. Yet the taboo continues to remind women that menstruation is a handicap. No wonder then that Snowden and Cristian[6] reported that mood changes prior to and during menstruation are directly related to the amount and duration of the bleeding episode, with shorter bleeding episodes and lighter bleeding closely related to the absence of mood change and physical discomfort. Even if this link has physiologic components, cultural factors are clearly at play as well.

In 1981 the Tampax Corporation commissioned a large-scale study of attitudes toward menstruation in the United States.[19] This research, based on a survey of 1,034 Americans ranging in age from 14 to over 65 who were interviewed by telephone, found that most Americans are still reticent about discussing menstruation openly, and most believe that women experience a significant amount of stress during menstruation (Table 2-2). About half believe that menstruation is painful, and 87 percent think that women are particularly emotional when menstruating. A substantial minority believe that women cannot function as well at work when menstruating. Those who were most likely to perceive menstruation as restrictive were subjects in the youngest and the oldest age groups (14 to 17 and over 55 years of age).

Education has an important influence on attitudes toward menstruation. In contrast to some of the beliefs about impairment seen in the studies of broad segments of the population in the United States and other parts of the

TABLE 2-2.   SELECTED ITEMS FROM THE TAMPAX SURVEY

Item	Agree Strongly (%)	Tend to Agree (%)	Tend to Disagree (%)	Disagree Strongly (%)
Women are more emotional when they are menstruating	58	29	8	5
Women can function as well at work when they are menstruating	48	26	17	9
Menstruation does not affect a woman's ability to think	48	17	17	18
Women do not need to restrict physical activities while menstruating	44	26	20	10

(Data from The Tampax Report. Ruder, Finn, & Rotman, New York, 1981.)

world, Brooks et al.[20] found that college women saw menstruation as a way of keeping in touch with their bodies and that it reflected a recurring affirmation of womanhood. Although these women also found menstruation to be bothersome, they did not perceive it to be particularly debilitating. Similarly, in a comparison of mothers and their college student daughters, Golub and Donnolo (unpublished study) found that the daughters had significantly more positive attitudes toward menstruation than did their mothers.

ATTITUDES AND SYMPTOMS

There is a great deal of controversy about the relation between attitudes toward menstruation and symptoms of menstrual distress. Most studies have been correlational, but that has not stopped some investigators from speculating that women who have negative attitudes are more likely to have symptoms (psychosomatic effect). Few of the studies suggest the possibility that experiencing pain or other symptoms, or even simply having long episodes of bleeding, might influence a woman's attitudes (somatopsychic effect), although this hypothesis generally appeals to women who have symptoms.

Levitt and Lubin,[21] in a study of menstrual complaints and menstrual attitudes, found a correlation of 0.32 between menstrual complaints and unwholesome attitudes. In the absence of any data regarding cause, they concluded that attitude and personality are factors in the *etiology* of menstrual symptoms.

Other researchers have also suggested a link between psychological problems and menstrual symptoms.[22-26] Some of these studies have been criticized by a number of authors on methodologic grounds.[27-30] The evidence supporting a relation between personality and symptoms is certainly contradictory, with studies by Coppen and Kessel[31] and Hirt et al.,[32] among others, finding no correlation. Nevertheless, in an article discussing the *DSM-III*, painful menstruation is cited as an example of a disorder that might be placed in the category "psychological factors affecting physical condition," a conclusion that seems out of keeping with current knowledge.[33] Other work, particularly that looking at dysmenorrhea, failed to find a causal link between attitudes and symptoms.[34,35] Similarly, Goudsmit reviewed a number of studies and concluded that there is little evidence to support the view that premenstrual symptoms are influenced by attitudes.[36]

MENARCHEAL EXPERIENCES AND SYMPTOMS

Some researchers have suggested that menarcheal experiences, particularly a lack of preparation for menarche, lead to negative attitudes and the subsequent development of perimenstrual symptoms.[26,37,38] However, in at least three studies no significant relation was found between adequacy of preparation or early experiences with menstruation and the subsequent experience of menstrual symptoms.[39-41] Golub and Catalano[39] found no relation between attitudes and symptoms or between preparation for menstruation and symptoms. Woods et al.[41] did find attitudes to be moderately associated with symptoms, but these authors suggested that the attitudes are probably influenced by the symptoms rather than the other way around.

AGE AND PREMENSTRUAL SYMPTOMS

INCIDENCE

Until recently there was no clear definition of what has come to be known as the premenstrual syndrome. (Several researchers have now proposed criteria for PMS, and in 1982 the Food and Drug Administration (FDA) Advisory Review Panel on Miscellaneous Over-the-Counter Internal Drug Products defined PMS for drug evaluation purposes.) Thus the number and variety of symptoms included vary widely from one study to another, from one woman to another, and within the same woman from one cycle to another. At best, PMS can be characterized as a group of psychological, somatic, and behavioral symptoms that are of sufficient severity to interfere with some aspects of life and that appear with a consistent and predictable relation to menses. Physical complaints include headache, backache, painful breasts, and symptoms of water retention. Psychological complaints include depression, anxiety, irritability, lethargy, and aggressiveness.

Because there has been no accepted general definition of premenstrual syndrome, efforts to compare published data in order to determine the incidence or prevalence of premenstrual problems have often been unrewarding. Thus incidence rates of up to 95 percent among normal women are cited.[3,5,25,31,42-45] In a report of United States and European studies concerning the prevalence of premenstrual symptoms among adult women, the incidence of symptoms ranged from a low of 4 percent for fatigue to a high of 70 percent for irritability.[5] These authors also found that their estimates for many symptoms closely resembled those from other studies. However, when they restricted their attention to severe symptoms, as opposed to mild or moderate ones, their prevalence estimates were considerably lower.

What about the relation between age and premenstrual symptoms?

Lloyd was the first to write about the "midthirties syndrome."[13] He noted the relation between age and premenstrual symptoms, particularly irritability and depression, and pointed out that the model age seems to lie around the 35th year. However, few studies have included a direct look at the relation between age and symptoms in normal women.

It is particularly difficult to assess the relation between premenstrual symptoms and age because so few studies include women over the age of 30. Most studies are of college or nursing students, who are usually under age 25. Moreover, the other populations that have been studied vary greatly, including normal women, PMS patients, prisoners, and psychiatric patients.

Nevertheless, there is some support for the belief that moderate to severe premenstrual symptoms are more likely to occur during the thirties and forties.[3,7,8,10,11,14,15] Among patients with premenstrual complaints, the average age reported is during the thirties.[10,11,46]

The incidence of premenstrual symptoms seems to increase after adolescence. Widholm and Kantero[47] found that edematous symptoms tripled in 5 years, going from 4.8 percent at age 12 to 15.1 percent at age 17. These authors also found a higher incidence of premenstrual symptoms in mothers than in their daughters (76 percent for the mothers compared to 67 percent for the daughters).

Moos,[3] in a study of 700 women, compared subjects under 21 with those over 31 and found that the older women were significantly more likely to complain of symptoms during the premenstrual phase of the cycle. In regard to correlations between age and symptoms, Moos noted that the correlation coefficients were low, perhaps indicating that age is not important when explaining menstrual cycle symptoms. However, the women in Moos' sample were generally young, with a mean age of only 25.2 years.

Analyzing the WHO data, Golub found that 29 percent of the women under 24 reported a mood change prior to menstruation compared with 57 percent of the women over 24 ($n = 5,287$). This age-related difference is highly significant.

Kramp[10] found a 50 percent incidence of premenstrual symptoms in his sample of women ranging in age from 15 to 45. There was a peak in the incidence of premenstrual symptoms of about 23 percent among women 30 to 39 years of age and another peak of about 20 percent in those ages 20 to 24. Kramp also noted an incidence of 30 percent among a group of psychiatric patients between the ages of 35 and 39. He concluded that PMS is most common in the 30- to 40-year age group.

In a study of 145 normal women and psychiatric patients between the ages of 15 and 45, Rees[14] found an approximately 25 percent incidence of moderate premenstrual "tension"* among the women who were 15 to 24 years of age, rising to 31 percent in the 25- to 34-year-old age group. Severe premenstrual tension was considerably more likely to be found after age 24,

---

*"Premenstrual tension" was defined by Rees as nervous tension, irritability, anxiety, depression, and such physical symptoms as bloating, breast swelling and tenderness, and headaches.

with an incidence of 30 percent. Rees also found a higher incidence of premenstrual tension among the psychiatric patients. He observed that nearly 80 percent of patients with premenstrual tension started before age 35, and in some the symptoms became worse after childbirth. In another study of a group of patients suffering from severe premenstrual tension, Rees[15] again found an increase in incidence with increasing age. In this group the reported incidence was as follows: 15 to 24 years 8 percent; 25 to 34 years 56 percent; 35 to 44 years 36 percent.

Focusing on the effects of oral contraceptives in a sample of normal women aged 18 to 46, Andersch and Hahn[12] found that nonusers of oral contraceptives over the age of 25 had a significantly higher incidence of premenstrual symptoms. The incidence of irritability among nonusers of oral contraceptives over 25 was 80 percent, and about 40 percent experienced anxiety and sadness. In contrast, among the 18-year-old women the incidence of sadness and anxiety was only 20 percent, half as much.

Dalton,[7] who has been studying patients with premenstrual syndrome for many years, reported an increased incidence with increasing age among both childless and parous women. Again the incidence reached a peak of about 30 percent among women between the ages of 35 and 44.

SEVERITY OF SYMPTOMS

In addition to looking at the incidence of premenstrual symptoms, it is important to look at their severity. As noted earlier, Woods et al.[5] found that 2 to 8 percent of women experience disabling symptoms. A few studies permit comparison between the menstrual and premenstrual pain and negative affect scores of subjects of various ages on the Menstrual Distress Questionnaire.[3,8,9,48-50]

As shown in Table 2-3, the younger subjects experienced more pain during menstruation with mean scores of about 18 and 15. The older subjects, those 25 and above, had mean scores around 12.5. The PMS subjects reported more premenstrual pain, with mean scores of about 17. Moos reported a menstrual pain mean score of 12.59, which indicates mild symptoms; the higher

TABLE 2-3. MENSTRUAL DISTRESS QUESTIONNAIRE: PAIN SCALE SCORES

Study	Score (Mean)	
	Menstrual	Premenstrual
Golub & Harrington[9] age 15–16	17.84	13.96
Gruba & Rohrbaugh[48] age 17–23	14.85	11.70
Moos[50] age mean 25.2	12.59	10.13
Golub[8] age 30–45	12.56	11.56
Maddocks[49] age 30–45	12.67	16.94

TABLE 2-4.   MENSTRUAL DISTRESS QUESTIONNAIRE: NEGATIVE AFFECT SCORES

	Mean Score	
Study	Menstrual	Premenstrual
Golub & Harrington[9] age 15–16	17.66	14.66
Gruba & Rohrbaugh[48] age 17–23	22.15	20.08
Moos[50] age mean 25.2	15.79	16.96
Golub[8] age 30–45	14.77	19.71
Maddocks[49] age 30–45	18.33	25.41

scores would indicate moderately severe but not strong or disabling symptoms. Nevertheless, 11 percent of Moos's sample reported strong or severe menstrual cramps.

Table 2-4 focuses on Menstrual Distress Questionnaire Negative Affect scores. Here the differences between the menstrual and premenstrual scores are of interest. Negative affect is greatest during the menstrual phase of the cycle for the two younger groups, whereas it is greater during the premenstrual phase of the cycle in the two older groups and the PMS subjects. Moos reported a menstrual mean of about 16 and a premenstrual mean of about 17, which indicates that on the average women's symptoms of negative affect range from barely noticeable to mild. However, a number of Moos' subjects reported strong or severe symptoms of depression (9.5 percent), tension (9.2 percent), mood swings (9.6 percent), and irritability (13 percent).[50] Despite "severe" depression and "mood swings," Moos's subjects were all normal women, not psychiatric patients.

The use of standardized measures of depression and anxiety permits comparison with normative data and a more meaningful assessment of the magnitude of the premenstrual and menstrual mood changes. In 1976 Golub[8] studied a group of normal women over the age of 30 and demonstrated that a significant premenstrual mood change did indeed occur in this age group, but the magnitude of the change was small and sharply different from levels seen in psychiatric illness or in people reacting to unusual stress. In 1981 Golub and Harrington[9] used the same measures to assess depression and anxiety during the premenstrual and menstrual phases of the cycle in a group of high school students with a mean age of 15 to 16 years. No significant change in mood across cycle phase was found on the Depression Adjective Check List or the State-Trait Anxiety Inventory* in these young women, although the same tests had shown changes in the older group.

In 1983 and 1984 two studies were done using the same measures with

---

*The State-Trait Anxiety Inventory measures both state anxiety, a transitory emotional state, and trait anxiety or anxiety-proneness, which is a relatively stable personality characteristic.

TABLE 2-5.   DEPRESSION

Group	Depression Scores (Mean)	
Normal adult women[a]	7.80	
Depressed psychiatric patients[a]	16.03	
	Intermenstrual	Premenstrual
High school students[b]	8.82	8.93
Adult women[c]	6.84	9.30
PMS patients[d]	9.00	17.50

[a]Normative data from Lubin.[52]
[b]Data from Golub and Harrington.[9]
[c]Data from Golub.[8]
[d]Data from Goudsmit.[36]

TABLE 2-6.   ANXIETY

Group	State Anxiety Scores (Mean)	
College students[a]		
Unstressed	35.12	
During an examination	43.69	
Patients[a]		
Medical-surgical	42.68	
Neuropsychiatric depressive reaction	54.43	
	Intermenstrual	Premenstrual
High school students[b]	41.79	41.41
Adult women[c]	33.64	38.10
PMS patients		
Goudsmit[d]	35.00	55.00
Maddocks[e]	40.33	56.68

[a]Normative data from Spielberger et al.[54]
[b]Data from Golub and Harrington.[9]
[c]Data from Golub.[8]
[d]Data from Goudsmit[36]
[e]Data from Maddocks[49]

PMS patients. These women appeared to be quite different from the normal subjects discussed above. Goudsmit[36] focused on 20 outpatients attending a PMS research clinic at St. Thomas' Hospital in London. The women ranged in age between 24 and 45, with an average age of 34.4. Mean premenstrual Depression Adjective Check List (DACL) scores for these women were about 17.50, comparable to those of depressed psychiatric patients (Table 2-5). Premenstrual state anxiety scores averaged about 55, again comparable to those of psychiatric patients with a depressive reaction (Table 2-6).

Maddocks[49] studied 44 women with severe PMS. Subjects ranged in age from 20 to 45 years with a mean of 35 years. Critieria for inclusion in the study were strict and included

1. Premenstrual dysphoric symptoms for at least six preceding cycles
2. Moderate to severe physical and psychological premenstrual symptoms

15

3. Symptoms only during the premenstrual period with marked relief at onset of menses
4. Age between 18 and 45 years
5. Not pregnant
6. No hormonal contraception
7. Regular menses for six previous cycles
8. No psychiatric disorder

Premenstrual state anxiety was significantly higher than that of the intermenstrual or menstrual phases of the cycle (mean 56.68) and was comparable to that reported by Goudsmit[36] and by Steiner et al.,[51] who reported a mean of 55. Maddocks used the Beck Depression Inventory rather than the DACL. Therefore the depression scores of this sample are not directly comparable to the others. However, Maddocks found that these women were on average "moderately depressed premenstrually (mean 16.69), mildly depressed during menstruation (mean 10.35), and not depressed intermenstrually (mean 5.73)." These data indicate that symptoms persist during menstruation, and they underline the need to study women throughout the cycle, not just premenstrually. Once again, these findings are comparable to those of Goudsmit[36] and show that women with severe premenstrual changes differ from normal women on standard psychological measures of depression and anxiety. These differences seem to apply to women in any age group at any phase of the cycle.

SUMMARY AND CONCLUSIONS

The emphasis in this chapter has been on the relation between age and symptoms of perimenstrual distress. The research literature supports the perception of clinicians who have said that young women more often experience dysmenorrhea and negative affect during menstruation, whereas older women are more likely to complain of somatic and psychological symptoms prior to menstruation (premenstrual). There does seem to be an increase in both the incidence and magnitude of premenstrual negative affect with age. At this time there is no satisfactory explanation for why it is so. It might be related to hormonal or neurohormonal changes, to target organ changes, or perhaps to heightened sensitivity to perimenstrual body changes among older women. This age group may have more negative attitudes toward menstruation. Alternatively, more severe premenstrual symptoms might be related to greater stress in the lives of older women. Higher levels of stress have been reported to affect premenstrual tension, anxiety, and depression.[11]

What about the myth of menstrual impairment? What do the data show about the effects of menstruation on women's cognitive and work performance? In a survey of the literature on the effects of menstruation on cognitive and perceptual motor tasks, Sommer[30] found 11 studies showing menstrual cycle effects, with some showing better performance during the premenstrual or menstrual phase of the cycle. Sommer also found 18 studies showing no phase difference in performance. The tasks included everything from simple perceptual motor tasks, e.g., time estimation or digit symbol coding, to complex problem-solving and concept formation tests. Thus although there is a high incidence of mild to moderate premenstrual symptoms among all age groups, Sommer's review confirmed the findings of almost 50 years of research in this area. The menstrual cycle has no consistent demonstrable effect on cognitive tasks, work, or academic performance despite beliefs to the contrary that persist. It is imperative that these findings be made known so that research on this intriguing mind–body problem is not hampered by concerns that these syndromes reduce women's credibility as responsible and reliable workers.

REFERENCES

1. Bergsjo P, Jenssen H, Vellar O: Dysmenorrhea in industrial workers. Acta Obstet Gynecol Scand 54:255, 1975
2. Kessel N, Coppen A: The prevalence of common menstrual symptoms. Lancet 2:61, 1963
3. Moos R: The development of a menstrual distress questionnaire. Psychosom Med 30:853, 1968
4. Sobvzyk R: Dysmenorrhea, the neglected syndrome. J Reprod Med 25(4):198, 1980
5. Woods NF, Most A, Dery GK: Prevalence of perimenstrual symptoms. Am J Public Health 72:1257, 1982
6. Snowden R, Christian B: Patterns and Perceptions of Menstruation. St. Martin's Press, New York, 1983
7. Dalton K: The Premenstrual Syndrome. Charles C Thomas, Springfield, IL, 1964
8. Golub S: The magnitude of premenstrual anxiety and depression. Psychosom Med 38:4, 1976
9. Golub S, Harrington DM: Premenstrual and menstrual mood changes in adolescent women. J Pers Soc Psychol 5:961, 1981
10. Kramp J: Studies on the premenstrual syndrome in relation to psychiatry. Acta Psychiatr Scand 203:261, 1968
11. Abplanalp JM, Haskett R, Rose R: The premenstrual syndrome. Psychiatr Clin North Am 3:327, 1980
12. Andersch B, Hahn L: Premenstrual complaints. II. Influence of oral contraceptives. Acta Obstet Gynecol Scand 60:569, 1981
13. Lloyd TS: The mid-thirties syndrome. Va Med Monthly 90:51, 1963
14. Rees L: Psychosomatic aspects of the premenstrual tension syndrome. Br Med J 99:62, 1953
15. Rees L: The premenstrual tension syndrome and its treatment. Br Med J 1:1014, 1953
16. Wood C, Larsen L, Williams R: Social and psychological factors in relation to premenstrual tension and menstrual pain. Aust NZ J Obstet Gynaecol 19:111, 1979
17. Ford CS, Beach FA: Patterns of Sexual Behavior. Harper & Row, New York, 1951
18. Stephens WN: A cross-cultural study of menstrual taboos. p. 67. In Ford CS (ed): Cross-Cultural Approaches. HRAF Press, New Haven, 1967
19. The Tampax Report. Ruder, Finn, & Rotman, New York, 1981
20. Brooks J, Ruble DN, Clarke A: College women's attitudes and expectations concerning menstrual-related changes. Psychol Med 39:288, 1977

21. Levitt EE, Lubin B: Some personality factors associated with menstrual complaints and menstrual attitude. J Psychiatr Res 11:267, 1967
22. Berry C, McGuire FL: Menstrual distress and acceptance of sexual role. Am J Obstet Gynecol 114:83, 1972
23. Gough H: Personality factors related to reported severity of menstrual distress. J Abnorm Psychol 1:59, 1975
24. Israel SL: Menstrual Disorders and Sterility. Harper & Row, Evanston, IL, 1975
25. Paulson MJ: Psychological concomitants of premenstrual tension. Am J Obstet Gynecol 81:733, 1956
26. Shainess N: A re-evaluation of some aspects of femininity through a study of menstruation: a preliminary report. Compr Psychiatry 2:20, 1961
27. Gannon L: Evidence for a psychological etiology of menstrual disorders: a critical review. Psychol Rep 48:287, 1981
28. Parlee MB: Stereotypic beliefs about menstruation: a methodological note on the Moos Menstrual Distress Questionnaire and some new data. Psychosom Med 36:229, 1974
29. Ruble DN: Premenstrual symptoms: a reinterpretation. Science 197:291, 1977
30. Sommer B: How does menstruation affect cognitive competence and psychophysiological response? Women Health 8(2–3):53, 1983
31. Coppen A, Kessel N: Menstruation and personality. Br J Psych 109:711, 1963
32. Hirt M, Kurtz R, Ross WD: The relationship between dysmenorrhea and selected personality variables. Psychosomatics 8:350, 1967
33. Spitzer RL, Williams JBW, Skodol AE: DSM III: the major achievements and an overview. Am J Psych 137:151, 1980
34. Lawlor C, Davis A: Primary dysmenorrhea. J Adolesc Health Care 1:208, 1981
35. Stoltzman SM: Menstrual attitudes, beliefs, and symptom experiences of adolescent females, their peers, and their mothers. Paper presented at the meeting of the Society for Menstrual Cycle Research, San Francisco, 1983
36. Goudsmit EM: Psychological aspects of premenstrual symptoms. J Psychosom Obstet Gynecol 2:20, 1983
37. Brooks-Gunn J, Ruble D: Dysmenorrhea in adolescence. p. 251. In Golub S (ed): Menarche. Lexington Books, Lexington, MA, 1983
38. Garwood SB, Allen L: Self-concept and identified problem differences between pre- and postmenarcheal adolescents. J Clin Psychol. 35:528, 1979
39. Golub S, Catalano J: Recollections of menarche and women's subsequent experiences with menstruation. Women Health 8(1):49, 1983
40. Slade P, Jenner FA: Performance tests in different phases of the menstrual cycle. J Psychosom Res 24:5, 1980
41. Woods NF, Dery GK, Most A: Recollections of menarche, current menstrual attitudes, and perimenstrual symptoms. p. 87. In Golub S (ed): Menarche. Lexington Books, Lexington, MA, 1983
42. Ferguson JH, Vermillion MB: Premenstrual tension: two surveys of its prevalence and a description of the syndrome. Obstet Gynecol 9:615, 1957
43. Perr IN: Medical, psychiatric, and legal aspects of premenstrual tension. Am J Psych 115:211, 1958
44. Pennington WM: Meprobamate in premenstrual tension. JAMA 164:683, 1957
45. Sutherland H, Stewart I: A critical analysis of the premenstrual syndrome. Lancet 1:1180, 1965
46. Kashiwagi T, McClure JN Jr, Wetzel RD: Premenstrual affective syndrome and psychiatric disorder. Dis Nerv Syst 37:116, 1976

47. Widholm O, Kantero RL: Menstrual patterns of adolescent girls according to chronological and gynecological ages. Acta Obstet Gynecol Scand 50(4):19, 1971
48. Gruba GH, Rohrbaugh M: MMPI correlates of menstrual distress. Psychosom Med 37:265, 1975
49. Maddocks SE: The investigation of symptom response patterns on a sample of women with severe premenstrual syndrome. Master's thesis, Queen's University, Kingston, Ontario, Canada, 1984
50. Moos RH: Menstrual Distress Questionnaire Manual. Stanford University, Stanford, CA, 1977
51. Steiner M, Haskett RF, Carroll BJ: Premenstrual syndrome, the development of research, diagnostic criteria, and new rating scales. Acta Psychiatr Scand 62:177, 1980
52. Lubin B: Manual for the Depression Adjective Check Lists. Educational and Industrial Testing Service, San Diego, CA, 1967
53. Halbreich U, Endicott J: Classification of premenstrual syndromes. p. 243. In Friedman RC (ed): Behavior and the Menstrual Cycle. Marcel Dekker, New York, 1982
54. Spielberger CD, Gorsuch RL, Lushene RE: STAI Manual, Consulting Psychologists Press, Palo Alto, CA, 1970

3

Basic Research Perspective: Ovarian Hormone Influence on Brain Neurochemical Functions

Bruce S. McEwen

Because we cannot determine if the female rats used in basic research experiments actually experience any of the premenstrual syndromes as they are known in humans, this chapter reviews the effects of hormones on the brain at a fundamental level. It is hoped that it gives a basis for understanding the interactions that exist between ovarian hormones and brain function and sets the stage for a more sophisticated understanding of the variety of complex and enigmatic premenstrual syndromes.

The study of hormones and the brain is at the same time old and new. The old part refers to the fact that some of the first experiments in the field of endocrinology published in 1849 by Berthold[1] dealt with the effects of gonadal hormones on the brains of roosters. The field is new in that our conception of how nerve cells work and communicate with one another has finally reached the point where we can begin to incorporate the external hormonal signals into our understanding of this aspect of brain function.

NEURAL TRANSMISSION

Figure 3-1 indicates three progressively more complex views of neural transmission. The classic view that still exists in many textbooks is that nerve cells produce and release neurotransmitters that act on postsynaptic receptors and transfer the electrical signal to the receiving cell; in this view these transmitters can be excitatory or inhibitory (view I). We have begun to realize that this process is considerably more complex, however (view II). These synaptic terminals that release neural transmitters have presynaptic receptors that en-

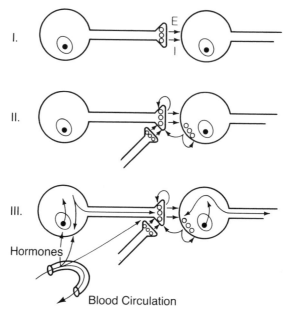

Fig. 3-1 Three progressively more complex views of the process of neurotransmission, showing in view III the influence of the hormones that reach the brain from the blood.

able them to monitor and respond to the transmitters they release and thereby modify the subsequent release of additional transmitters. Moreover, the presynaptic endings frequently possess receptors for other transmitters produced and released by other neurons in the vicinity. Through this lateral communication at the level of presynaptic nerve endings chemicals produced by other nerve endings have the ability to influence the release of chemicals from these presynaptic endings. In addition, we know that in a number of instances the postsynaptic structures that are called dendrites produce and release transmitters that act upon themselves as well as influence presynaptic neurotransmitter release. Thus the process of neural transmission is not entirely a one-way process but can be at least a two-way process in that the postsynaptic cell can influence what the presynaptic neuron is doing.

Finally (Fig. 3-1, view III), blood vessels serving the brain carry hormonal signals produced in other parts of the body and can act directly at nerve endings and indirectly through the cell body and the cell nucleus. A blood-borne hormone, such as epinephrine, is also produced locally by neurons as a neurotransmitter. Therefore as a hormone it may have access to sites not available as a neurotransmitter or vice versa. Other hormones, e.g., ACTH and prolactin, are known to enter at least selective regions of the brain and influence nerve cell activity by cell surface receptors. Steroidal hormones actually enter nerve cells and cause the cell nucleus to activate or suppress the expression of genes, many of which are involved in producing the enzymes, neurotransmitters, structural proteins, and receptors that make nerve cells work. This

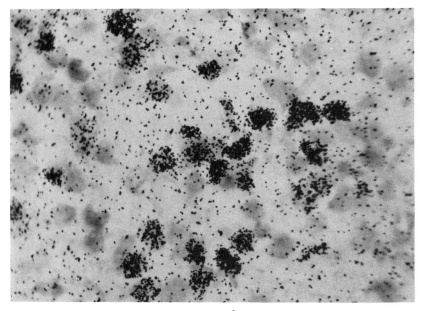

Fig. 3-2 Group of neurons that concentrate ³H-estrogen in the hypothalamus of a 3-day-old rat, showing the clustering of estrophilic nerve cells in specific places in the brain. (Autoradiography by J. Gerlach. × 725.)

chapter is a discussion of how gonadal hormones, primarily estradiol and to some extent progesterone, operate in the brain.

Figure 3-2 shows an autoradiogram of nerve cells that have accumulated radioactive estradiol. It shows that the nerve cells that have receptors for the female hormone estradiol are clustered in groups.[2] The figure represents the ventromedial nucleus of the hypothalamus, and the black dots are the silver grains produced by the radioactive decay from the tissue exposing adjacent film. This process is called *autoradiography*. In the rat these estradiol-concentrating nerve cells occur in discrete clusters scattered throughout the brain but are found in highest concentrations within the hypothalamus, in the preoptic area, and more laterally in the amygdala.

ESTROGEN EFFECTS

It is clear that estrogen comes to the brain and is picked up and returned by specific cell receptors. What is it doing in these cells? What does estrogen do to brain function? Using the technique of iontophoresis, in which estrogens are placed on nerve cells in the hypothalamus, it is possible to show rapid and direct changes in electrical activity produced by estradiol.[3] The natural estrogen 17β-estradiol hemisuccinate is effective, whereas 17α-estradiol hemisuccinate does not produce these effects, indicating that the brain displays a stereoselectivity similar to the requirement for biologic potency of estradiol elsewhere (e.g., in the uterus). In the brain it is clear that this hormonal signal is translated into a direct nerve cell response.

The principal mode of steroid hormone action involves entering the cell; and if that cell has produced as part of its differentiation a specific receptor protein, it interacts with that receptor protein and then moves into the cell nucleus. The receptor–hormone complex then interacts with the genome to activate or suppress the expression of specific genes in terms of messenger RNA production and subsequent protein synthesis. This estrogen activity can be described in terms of acetylcholine, an important neurotransmitter, and then tyrosine hydroxylase, which is a rate-limiting enzyme for the production of the catecholamines, epinephrine and norepinephrine, from tyrosine. Estrogen treatment of a female rat results in a nearly twofold induction of choline acetyltransferase activity in one of five cholinergic cell groupings within the basal forebrain (Fig 3-3).[4] The basal forebrain is the area of the brain that has been implicated in Alzheimer's disease. Thus we can show highly localized effects of estrogens in inducing important neurotransmitter-related enzymes. Induction or increased level of synthesis is not the only estrogen effect in nerve tissue. We showed that estrogen treatment for a number of days *decreased* the activity of tyrosine hydroxylase (TH) in the hypothalamus (Fig.

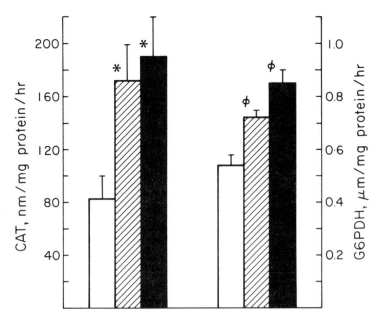

Fig. 3-3 Effect of estradiol on activity of choline acetyltransferase (CAT) in the nucleus of the horizontal limb of the diagonal band of Broca and on the activity of glucose-6-phosphate dehydrogenase (G6PDH) in the pituitary. The effects of 6 hours (hatched bars) and 24 hours (black bars) of estradiol treatment were measured at 24 hours after beginning hormone treatment of ovariectomized rats. (Luine VN, McEwen BS: Sex differences in cholinergic diagonal band nuclei in the rat preoptic area. Neuroendocrinology 36:475, 1983, S. Karger AG, Basel.)

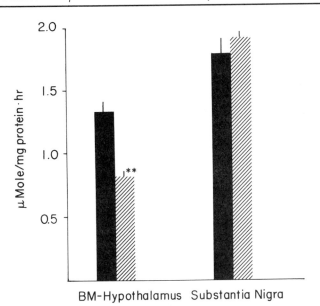

Fig. 3-4 Effect of 7 days of estradiol treatment on the activity of tyrosine hydroxylase in the basal hypothalamus and substantia nigra of ovariectomized rats. (Luine VN, McEwen BS, Black IB: Effect of 17β-estradiol on hypothalamic tyrosine hydroxylase activity. Brain Res 120:188, 1977.

3-4).[5] As noted, TH manufactures catecholamines from tyrosine. Furthermore, the effect is anatomically specific. There is no effect of estrogen treatment in the superior cervical ganglion or in a number of other brain regions, including the substantia nigra. The basal hypothalamus includes nerve endings from other catecholamine systems in the brain in addition to a small group of tuberoinfundibular neurons with their cell bodies in this part of the brain. How specific is the estrogen effect in the hypothalamus? One way of determining if there is a more profound effect of estrogen treatment on these cell bodies that accumulate estradiol is to actually measure the messenger RNA for tyrosine hydroxylase, which has been done in a collaborative study with Blum and Roberts at Columbia University. In this experiment, using a cDNA probe developed by Chikarashi, we were able to show that after estrogen priming there is a decrease in the rate of transcription of the tyrosine hydroxylase gene using a rate transcription runoff assay. The rate of transcription decreases within 20 to 60 minutes of estrogen treatment to practically zero. In contrast, using a cDNA probe for the anterior pituitary to look at prolactin, which is a pituitary hormone influenced by estrogens, the same estrogen treatment results in a marked increase in the transcription of the prolactin gene within 60 minutes. Obviously, the effects of estradiol on gene transcription and enzyme induction can be both positive and negative in discrete areas of the brain.

Another important aspect of steroid hormone action involves their influence on neurotransmitter receptors. There are biosynthetic and degradative enzymes for neurotransmitters as well as receptors for neurotransmitters. Together these three gene products play an important role in regulating the excitability and electrical activity of nerve cells.

Several laboratories have developed techniques for performing quantitative autoradiography of neurotransmitter receptors. Basically the method employs fresh frozen sections that are labeled with specific radioactive hormones or drugs. To assay the degree of receptor binding, the sections are exposed to a highly tritium-sensitive film. At the end of several months the autoradiograms are developed and stained. A densitometer is used to measure the intensity of labeling in various experimental manipulations, e.g., estrogen effects on neurotransmitter receptor levels. Studies by Johnson et al.[6] examined guinea pig brain (Fig. 3-5). Estrogen treatment, which enhances sexual behavior in the female guinea pig, leads to a 30 percent increase in the binding of tritiated paraaminoclonidine to α_2-adrenergic receptors in the preoptic area.

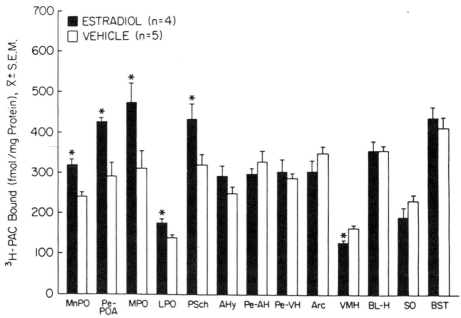

Fig. 3-5 Effect of estradiol treatment for several days on levels of α_2-adrenergic receptors in various estrogen-sensitive areas of hypothalamus and preoptic area of ovariectomized guinea pig. MnPO = median preoptic nucleus. Pe-POA = preoptic periventricular area. MPO = medial preoptic area. LPO = lateral preoptic area. PSch = preoptic suprachiasmatic area. AHY = anterior hypothalamic area. Pe-AH = periventricular nucleus of the anterior hypothalamus. Pe-VH-periventricular area of the ventral hypothalamus. Arc = arcuate hypothalamic nucleus. VMH = ventromedial hypothalamic nucleus. BL-H = basolateral hypothalamic area. SO = supraoptic hypothalamic nucleus. BST = bed nucleus of the stria terminalis. (Johnson AE, Nock B, McEwen BS, Feder HH: Estradiol modulation of α_2- noradrenergic receptors of guinea pig brain assessed by tritium-sensitive film autoradiography. Brain Res 336:153, 1985.)

α_2-receptors respond to catecholamines such as norepinephrine, which is a neurotransmitter produced by nerve cells in the brain stem, which distributes its projections over the entire forebrain. There are a number of other brain areas that are also estrogen-sensitive (e.g., the arcuate nucleus) which show no change in α-adrenergic receptors after estrogen priming, and then there is a slight but significant decrease in the ventromedial nucleus of the hypothalamus, which controls feminine sexual behavior in rats and guinea pigs. Clearly the response of estrogen-concentrating areas of the brain to the hormone is diverse. Not every estrogen-sensitive brain area shows the same response to the hormone.

SEROTONIN-1 RECEPTOR SYSTEM

Another receptor system, the serotonin-1 receptor system in the rat, is also sensitive to estradiol.[7] Serotonin is a transmitter produced by cells in the base of the brain that project to the forebrain. We studied the effects of estrogen priming in both male and female rats on the level of serotonin-1 receptors.[8] In Figure 3-6 the results are expressed, for comparative purposes between male and female rats, as percent of control, so that an increase (above the line) represents an increase in receptor level and a decrease (below the line) represents a decrease in receptor level. The open bars, which represent the female rats exposed in vivo to estradiol for several days, show that in the

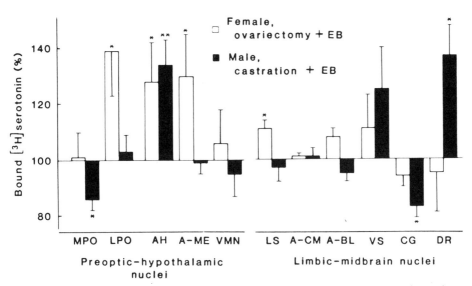

Fig. 3-6 Effects of estrogen treatment on levels of serotonin-1 receptors in various brain areas of gonadectomized male and female rats. MPO = medial preoptic area. LPO = lateral preoptic area. AH = anterior hypothalamus. A-ME = arcuate-median eminence. VMN = ventromedial nucleus. LS = lateral septum. A-CM = amygdala, corticomedial. A-BL = amygdala, basolateral. VS = ventral subiculum. CG = midbrain central gray. DR = dorsal raphe. (Fischette CT, Biegon A, McEwen BS: Sex differences in serotonin-1 receptor binding in rat brain. Science 222:333, 1983. Copyright 1983 by the American Association for the Advancement of Science.)

lateral preoptic area, the anterior hypothalamus, the arcuate median eminence, and the lateral septum—all of which have estrogen-sensitive neurons—there is increased serotonin receptor binding. We examined male rats because we know that male brains have estrogen receptors and that estradiol is an important hormone in the male rat. In fact, testosterone, the male hormone, is converted in certain regions of the brain to estradiol and interacts with estrogen receptors, making estrogen an important hormone in the male as well as the female brain. Yet we know that there are important structural and behavioral differences between male and female rats that point to inherent differences in the brain that are not simply related to which circulating hormone is present. When estradiol is given to castrated male rats there is only one area of the male brain that responds the same way: the anterior hypothalamus. It shows an induction of serotonin-1 receptors after estrogen treatment in both male and female rats. Other areas of the brain respond differently. Medial preoptic area serotonin-1 receptors decrease in male rats after estrogen, whereas they do not change in the female rat. There is no male response in the lateral preoptic area and the lateral septum or in the arcuate nucleus-median eminence region. Moreover, in response to estrogen there is in the male rat a significant decrease that was not found in the female rat in the midbrain central gray and a significant increase in the dorsal raphé nucleus, which again was not seen in the female. These results reinforce the idea that it is more than just the circulating hormones that are present in the male and female brains. Rather, there are intrinsic differences in the way the brain responds to hormones.

ROLE OF PROGESTERONE

Progesterone is an important ovarian hormone involved in modifying, amplifying, or inhibiting many of the effects of estrogens. It is an important synergistic hormone in the activation of sexual behavior in rats and other species. It also acts synergistically with estradiol in amplifying the luteinizing hormone (LH) surge, which causes ovulation. Under certain circumstances, it also is thought to help terminate some of these events and to be inhibitory. Thus there may be sequential or concurrent inhibition by elevated progesterone levels as well as the synergistic facilitation of estrogen-dependent responses.

The key connection between estrogens and progestins is that there is estrogen induction of progesterone receptor sites in certain areas of the brain as well as in the pituitary and uterus. Figure 3-7 shows uptake of a tritium-labeled progestin in the ventromedial nucleus region of an adult female rat. The infrahuman primate brain of the rhesus monkey contains estrogen and estrogen-inducible progestin receptors in much the same distribution as we see in the rat brain.[9] We therefore believe that it is probably a feature of the human brain as well.

Figure 3-8 shows results of a study in which we measured biochemically

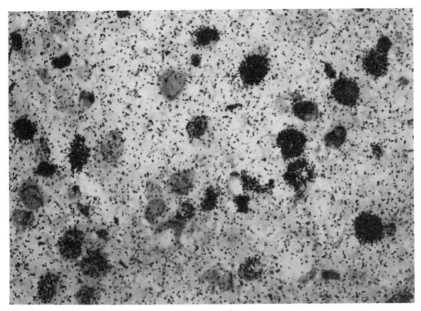

Fig. 3-7 Group of neurons that concentrate a ³H-labeled synthetic progestogenic steroid in the hypothalamus of an estrogen-primed rat. (Autoradiography by J. Gerlach. × 725.)

the induction of progestin receptor sites in various estrogen-sensitive brain regions.[10] Many of the same brain areas that we have been talking about for neurotransmitter receptors and enzyme inductions show progestin receptor induction. However, there are some estrogen-sensitive brain areas, e.g., medial amygdala and bed nucleus of the stria terminalis, which have estrogen receptors but show little if any induction of progesterone receptors by estradiol. Thus, again, the regulatory phenotype is highly diversified, and there is no single, absolute phenotype for any given estrogen-sensitive neuron, including the induction of these progesterone receptors.

Compared to estradiol, there is little knowledge about what progesterone does to the brain. Luine and Rhodes[11] observed in a number of hypothalamic areas of the female rat brain (incidentally, it may not be the same in the male brain) that estrogen priming for several days causes monoamine oxidase (MAO) levels to decrease. MAO is an enzyme important in the degradation of serotonin and catecholamines. MAO inhibitors are among the drugs that are used for modifying behavioral states of animals and people. The increase or decrease of MAO levels can have profound effects on mood and other aspects of behavior. Estrogens cause a decrease of type A MAO; if progesterone is then given, there is a rapid increase in MAO activity (Fig. 3-9). This reaction is an example of how progesterone treatment reverses the effect of the estrogen priming. If the MAO activity increases suddenly, it may cause a rapid degradation of monoamines. In contrast, the estrogen priming, by decreasing

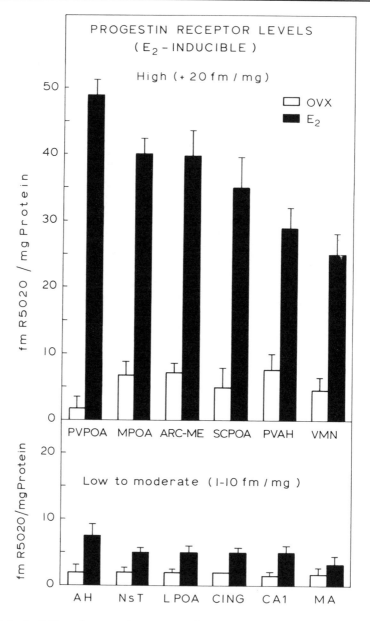

Fig. 3-8 Inducibility of progestin receptors by estrogen treatment of ovariectomized rats. PVPOA = periventricular preoptic area. MPOA = medial preoptic area. ARC-ME = arcuate nucleus-median eminence. SCPOA = suprachiasmatic preoptic area. PVAH = periventricular anterior hypothalamus. VMN = ventromedial nucleus. AH = anterior hypothalamus. NsT = bed nucleus of stria terminalis. LPOA = lateral preoptic area. CING = cingulate cortex. CA1 = hippocampus Ammon's horn. MA = medial amygdala. (Parsons B, Rainbow TC, MacLusky N, McEwen BS: Progestin receptor levels in rat hypothalamic and limbic nuclei. J Neurosci 2:1446, 1982 © Society for Neuroscience.)

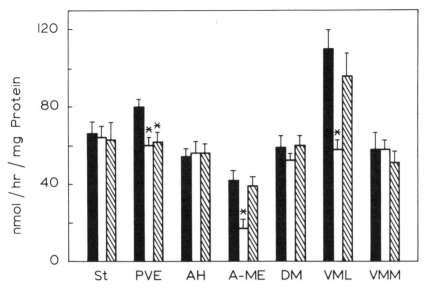

Fig. 3-9 Monoamine oxidase activity is shown after treatment of ovariectomized rats with estradiol for 3 days (open bar) and estradiol followed by progesterone for 1 hour (hatched bars). St = striatum. PVE = periventricular preoptic area. AH = anterior hypothalamus. A-ME = arcuate nucleus-median eminence. DM = dorsomedial nucleus. VML, VMM = ventromedial nucleus, lateral and medial, respectively. (Luine VN, Rhodes JC: Gonadal hormone regulation of MAO and other enzymes in hypothalamic areas. Neuroendocrinology 36:235, 1983, S. Karger AG, Basel.)

MAO, tends to cause the amines to build up slowly. Thus the sequential presence of estradiol followed by progesterone might have fundamental effects on levels of monoamines through this mechanism.

One interesting fact is that this effect of progesterone on MAO occurs when the animal has been previously exposed to estradiol. Secondly, whereas many of the effects of estradiol are blocked by a protein synthesis inhibitor, this particular effect of progesterone is not. Thus it is possible that there are direct membrane-mediated and direct enzymatic effects of steroids such as progesterone, which may in turn depend on the prior genomic actions of estradiol. Again, all of these events take place within highly localized parts of the brain. There is no single generalization for all estrogen- or progestin-sensitive areas of the brain. Certainly there are many parts of the brain that do not appear to be sensitive to hormones at all.

Figure 3-10 outlines another way of looking at hormone action.[12] It shows the nerve cell body with its nucleus and nucleolus. Hormones induce a change of gene expression leading to protein synthesis and transport of these newly synthesized proteins into the postsynaptic dendritic side or to the presynaptic side. Hormones may also have direct actions on nerve cell membranes, although these effects are limited in scope and duration, and may depend on genomic action of the same or different hormones.

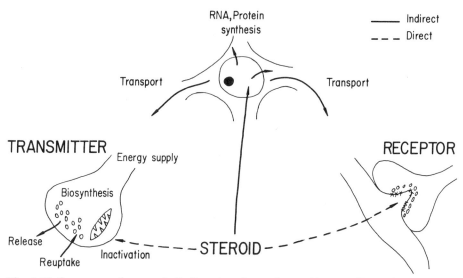

Fig. 3-10 Summary of genomic (indirect) and membrane (direct) effects of steroids on nerve cell function. (McEwen BS, Krey LC, Luine VN: Steroid hormone action in the neuroendocrine system: when is the genome involved? p. 255. In Reichlin S, Baldessarine RJ, Martin JB (eds): The Hypothalmus. Raven Press, New York, 1978.)

SUMMARY

Hormones such as estradiol and progesterone do affect the brain directly. The receptors and the effects of hormones through them are highly localized within hormone-sensitive, receptor-containing areas of the brain. They are also highly diverse. Various features of neurochemistry related to neural transmission appear to be altered through a genomic mechanism, i.e., the induction, or suppression, of genes related to biosynthetic and degradative enzymes for neurotransmitters as well as genes for neurotransmitter receptors. These genomic hormone effects can be long-lasting, i.e., on the order of hours and days or even weeks in some cases. There are also rapid membrane-mediated effects of estrogens and perhaps of progestins, which have a much shorter latency and duration.

The male and the female brains have subtle but nevertheless important structural and functional differences, including differences in the effects produced by gonadal hormones on localized or chemical functions. Yet the male brain also has estrogen receptors, and estradiol is an important hormone as a product of the local aromatization of testosterone in certain parts of the brain. Thus it must be borne in mind that men may be influenced psychologically and neurologically by their hormones, albeit in a different way from women.

Because mechanisms exist in the brain for it to respond to circulating hormones during estrus, or in the case of humans the menstrual cycle, this fact clearly can have important implications for the behavioral state and for the response to medications and psychotropic drugs.[13] Such drugs are administered to influence neurotransmitter systems and alter mood or neurologic states, and their ability to do so may at the same time be affected by circulating hormones.

REFERENCES

1. Berthold AA: Transplantation der Hoden. Arch Anat Physiol Will Med 16:42, 1849
2. Gerlach JL, McEwen BS, Toran-Allerand CD, Friedman WJ: Perinatal development of estrogen receptors in mouse brain assessed by radioautography, nuclear isolation and receptor assay. Dev Brain Res 11:7, 1983
3. Kelly MJ, Moss RL, Dudley CA, Fawcett CP: The specificity of the response of preoptic-septal area neurons to estrogen: 17β-estradiol vs 17β-estradiol and the response of extrahypothalamic neurons. Exp Brain Res 30:43, 1977
4. Luine VN, McEwen BS: Sex differences in cholinergic diagonal band nuclei in the rat preoptic area. Neuroendocrinology 36:475, 1983
5. Luine VN, McEwen BS, Black IB: Effect of 17β-estradiol on hypothalamic tyrosine hydroxylase activity. Brain Res 120:188, 1977
6. Johnson AE, Nock B, McEwen BS, Feder HH: Estradiol modulation of α_2-noradrenergic receptors in guinea pig brain assessed by tritium-sensitive film autoradiography. Brain Res 336:153, 1985
7. Biegon A, Fischette C, Rainbow TC, McEwen BS: Serotonin-1 modulation by estrogen in discrete brain nuclei. Neuroendocrinology 35:287, 1982
8. Fischette CT, Biegon A, McEwen BS: Sex differences in serotonin-1 receptor binding in rat brain. Science 222:333, 1983
9. MacLusky N, Lieberburg I, Krey LC, McEwen BS: Progesterone receptors in the brain and pituitary of a primate, the bonnet monkey (Macaca radiata). Endocrinology 106:185, 1980
10. Parsons B, Rainbow TC, MacLusky N, McEwen BS: Progestin receptor levels in rat hypothalamic and limbic nuclei. J Neurosci 2:1446, 1982
11. Luine VN, Rhodes JC: Gonadal hormone regulation of MAO and other enzymes in hypothalamic areas. Neuroendocrinology 36:235, 1983
12. McEwen BS, Krey LC, Luine VN: Steroid hormone action in the neuroendocrine system: when is the genome involved? p. 255. In Reichlin S, Baldessarini RJ, Martin JB (eds): The Hypothalmus, Raven Press, New York, 1978
13. Hamilton J, Parry B: Sex-related differences in clinical drug response: implications for women's health. J Am Med Wom Assoc 38:126, 1983

4
Toward a Clinical Research Perspective

Jean A. Hamilton
Sheryle W. Alagna

There has been a strong resurgence of clinical research interest in menstrual cycle-related mood and behavior changes. One approach to increasing our understanding of the menstrual cycle in humans is the study of estrous cycles in various animals. Despite the fact that the estrous cycle has somewhat different biologic characteristics in different animals, these physiologic processes have been shown to parallel aspects of the human menstrual cycle. Animal-based models are undoubtedly applicable and have advanced our knowledge of steroid hormone action on the brain. However, the assumptions underlying these approaches are limiting precisely because they do not address special aspects of having humans as research subjects. The goal of this chapter is to address this concern conceptually and empirically.

HUMANS AS RESEARCH SUBJECTS: SPECIAL FEATURES

There are advantages and disadvantages to conducting animal research compared to human research. The most obvious is that whereas animal research affords more control over experimental variables, clinical scientists are confronted with the actual complexity of human functioning; what clinicians gain is the opportunity to explore what is fully human about our lives.

Regardless of whether they are accurate, reductionistic assumptions about the regulation of behavior appear to be more workable in animals than in humans. Although much animal-based research has assumed direct biologic effects on behavior and situation-independent and cognitively indepen-

The opinion or assertions contained herein are the private ones of the authors and are not to be construed as official or reflecting the views of the Department of Defense or the Uniformed Services University of the Health Sciences.

dent laws of functioning, McClintock[1] and others have shown that such effects are not context-free even in animals.[1,2]

The cerebral cortex is a major contributor to behavioral variability. Because rodents evidence less cortical development than people, we expect animal-based studies with rodents to reveal comparatively less modulation of innate behavioral programming by means of cortical inhibition. However, within the range of normal human functioning, scientists observe highly modulated and variable behaviors. As shown by Ruble,[3] an adequate clinical perspective on the human menstrual cycle must recognize the conceptual and methodologic implications of such observations.

The actual conduct of clinical research on the menstrual cycle should reflect what most distinguishes human from animal research: the study of a subject who is thinking and self-reflective. That is, clinical scientists study women who variously conceptualize, modify, and report on their own experience. Hamilton et al.[4] have shown that cognitive approaches to menstrual cycle research provide a unique window on processes that may modify or mediate the effects of substance changes on symptomatology.

Many clinical scientists are primarily concerned with the application of basic science knowledge to diagnosis and treatment. Biomedical models for applied, clinical research share certain assumptions with animal-based models; for example, both assume powerful, direct effects, apart from situational and cognitive influences. Perhaps this assumption arises, in part, from a clinical focus on pathologic conditions, where normal functioning is so disrupted that modifying processes are, or appear to be, negligible.

Although biomedically oriented diagnostic and treatment studies have their place—one that is critically important—we must not overlook the fundamental difference between trying to understand something and trying to change it.[5] These two concerns are in constant competition: for the time and attention of researchers in the actual conduct of research, and for funding priority. Without a balance between efforts aimed at understanding and at application, we bias our fund of knowledge, however unintentionally, by omission.[6-8]

ARE SELECTION CRITERIA PREMATURE FOR THE GENERIC MENSTRUAL CYCLE STUDY?

In 1983 the National Intitute of Mental Health (NIMH) sponsored a conference aimed at establishing research guidelines for clinical studies of the menstrual cycle. The conference recommended that subjects meet the following criteria:

1. A marked change of about 30 percent in the intensity of symptoms measured intermenstrually, from cycle days 5 to 10, compared to that premenstrually, during the 6-day interval prior to menses
2. Documentation of these changes for at least two consecutive cycles

Although these guidelines are not meant to be universal "rules," the intent was to help shape the field by increasing the comparability of studies. A major focus was recommendations for selection criteria for the generic menstrual cycle study. More uniform and rigorous criteria increase homogeneity in subject populations and have particular merit for diagnostic, neuroendocrine, and treatment studies. For example, we found symptomatic group differences in plasma β-endorphin for a preselected, carefully screened population *only* when groups were defined by symptom changes in the actual cycle studied[9]; whereas global groupings were generally unrevealing (Hamilton and Alagna, unpublished data).

Are biomedically oriented or treatment studies the norm; and if so, should they be? The answer to the first question is yes, at least among psychiatric researchers, but we are concerned that this situation is far from optimal. In fact, we believe that some of the current recommendations for uniformity in menstrual cycle research are premature,* tending to foreclose research aimed at understanding symptomatology and sources of variability in favor of studies that diagnose or treat it.

Our purpose is not to critique these models conceptually or to offer alternative guidelines, which Koeske[10] and others[11] have already accomplished. Instead, we use data from a clinical study begun at NIMH to illustrate some of the actual uses and misuses of selection criteria. We believe that one of the goals of a clinical research perspective is to clarify the applicability of these selection criteria to the conduct of different types of menstrual cycle research.

We begin with a reexamination of proposals that focus on confirming symptoms or a menstrually linked syndrome by documenting changes in concurrent self-ratings. In order to provide a context for evaluating the use of multiple types and sources of measurement, we explore parallels between findings in menstrual cycle and affective disorders research. Finally, we document the utility of strategies aimed at the clarification of symptoms and sources of variance, rather than simple confirmation.

USES AND MISUSES OF SELECTION CRITERIA: CONCEPTUALIZING THE CONCORDANCE BETWEEN TYPES AND SOURCES OF MEASUREMENT IN MENSTRUAL CYCLE RESEARCH

Useful selection criteria have been proposed for the inclusion of subjects in menstrual cycle research[12-14]; also, the NIMH recommendations (S. Blumenthal, in preparation) have been cited by several investigators.[15,16] Because some of these criteria reflect and reinforce biomedically oriented models for research, however, they are likely to be reified and unintentionally overused.

---

*Recent debate have focused on a menstrual cycle-related psychiatric diagnosis, late luteal phase dysphoric disorder (LLDD).[9a,9b]

Rubinow and his colleagues[14] have proposed that the "existence of the premenstrual syndrome should be prospectively confirmed before a woman's entry into studies." These investigators assume that an arbitrary level of change in an isolated symptom such as "depressed mood" is adequate to "confirm or disprove" the existence of a premenstrual syndrome—or the fluctuation of mood "symptoms"—when assessed prospectively by longitudinal, concurrent self-ratings. Because these investigators do not address the generalizability of this criterion, it appears that they intend it to be used generically, for menstrual cycle studies at large.

In contrast, we believe that there are pros and cons to the application of this proposal to different kinds of menstrual cycle research, where it is clearly most suitable to biomedically oriented diagnostic and treatment studies. We are also concerned about the tendency to conceptualize concurrent self-ratings as "confirming or disproving" global self-perceptions about symptomatology, or a syndrome. An alternative to viewing these various types of information as competing is to see them as complementary. From this perspective, examining global self-reports of symptomatology in the context of other sources of information (e.g., observer rating, concurrent self-ratings) clarifies the meaning of women's experiences.

Several lines of evidence suggest that the concordance between various measures may enhance our understanding of menstrual cycle-related symptomatology. For subjects with globally, self-identified symptomatology, we found a mixed pattern of concordance between concurrent self and observer ratings. As shown in Figure 4-1, subject A would be considered disproved by the criteria discussed above because there is no premenstrual peak in her concurrent ratings of depression; yet her concurrent, "on–off" reports of having premenstrual syndrome (PMS), which typically involved observable symptoms such as depression, fatigue, and swelling, were positive in this cycle, as were those of a family observer (F). This example raises questions about the processes of self-perception involved in these reports and about simple conceptualizations of confirmation.

Although self and nursing observer ratings were concordant for "swelling," both sources indicated a midcycle rather than a premenstrual peak. Observer ratings were nonconcordant with the concurrent self-reports of a midcycle peak in fatigue. Although the observer ratings indicated a premenstrual peak in depression, tending to corroborate the subject's "on–off" ratings, these observer ratings actually lagged behind the midcycle peak in the concurrent depression self-ratings.

Other investigators have found that some women who report only premenstrual symptoms actually show two peaks, including one that occurs at midcycle[14,17]; in our clinical study, 57 percent of the self-identified highly symptomatic PMS women also showed a midcycle elevation for pain compared to 0 percent of the low symptom group. Perhaps the onset of menstruation provides such a salient marker for these experiences that premenstrual symptoms are preferentially encoded and recalled. Alternatively, there may

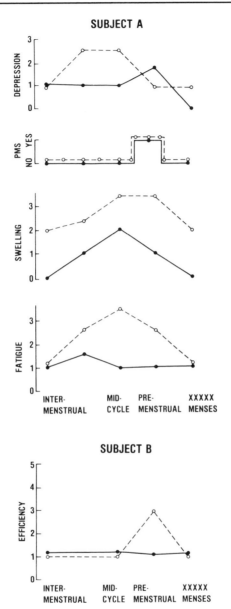

Fig. 4-1 (°——°) Averaged self ratings on the Moos (subscales or item). (•——•) Averaged observer ratings on pertinent items from the Steiner et al. scale.

be a lag between the midcycle peak in changes and the awareness or encoding of these experiences.

Self and observer ratings of another subject (B, Fig. 4-1) illustrate a different pattern. In this case changes in efficiency were not remembered to be salient to the subject's experience of PMS,[6] although she showed a clear premenstrual increase in symptomatology on this scale; furthermore, an observer failed to report changes specific to this time period, although his ratings did show variability across time.

OBJECTIVE MEASURES

Similarly, self-ratings of a premenstrual increase in fluid retention were not highly concordant with repeated measurements of weight.[18,19] Global reports of decreased performance premenstrually were not supported by concurrent objective measures of functioning in most women.[20] We have reported a discrepancy between concurrent self-ratings of concentration and actual measures of sustained attention in women with self-identified PMS.[4] These and other observations[21] led us to the hypothesis that some women may experience altered self-perceptions premenstrually; if so, these discrepancies may prove useful as tools for clarifying possible menstrual cycle effects on information processing, as they may be related to the initiation or modification of symptoms.[21a]

PARALLELS WITH RESEARCH ON AFFECTIVE DISORDERS

Research on affective disorders has clearly been advanced by the use of diagnostic criteria. However, psychiatric epidemiologists have not inferred that a depressive syndrome is confirmed merely by asking subjects to rate themselves on the single item of depression; instead, research on affective disorders has used rating scales, with multiple items employed for standardization.

In addition to using multi-item inventories, investigators have gathered measurements from a variety of sources. For depressives, Paykel and his colleagues[22] found only moderate concordance between self-reports and observer ratings. Mazure and her colleagues at Yale have begun to clarify the reliability of specific items on a modified Hamilton depression rating scale, as well as their observability, establishing the reliability and validity of a symptom inventory designed to assess depression (unpublished observations). This kind of careful work is needed in order to ensure that we are using reliable and valid measures in a given population, an issue that has been neglected in research on the menstrual cycle.

The discrepancy between global, retrospective vs. concurrent self-reports and objective performance measures has also been observed in a variety of populations. For example, female medical students, a group at increased risk for depression, are more likely to perceive themselves as performing inadequately compared to their male peers, despite the adequacy of their actual performance.[23,24] It is also well known that in depressed patients a gap is sometimes observed between the onset of improvement that is apparent to observers and that perceived by the patient.

There is increasing interest among researchers studying affective disorders in whether information processing alterations or discrepancies may be critical to understanding depression. It has been shown that certain subgroups remember their depressive symptoms more accurately than do others. For example, women are more likely than men to recognize or to remember and retrospectively report depression[25] and psychic distress.[26] As we have already demonstrated, these considerations are pertinent to understanding depressive mood changes that occur, or are conceptualized as occurring, premenstrually.

UTILITY OF HUMAN-BASED RESEARCH ON THE MENSTRUAL CYCLE: CLARIFICATION OF SYMPTOMS AND SOURCES OF VARIANCE

Even if there were agreement on how to "confirm" cases of PMS, do we really want to limit ourselves to this subject population? When answering this question, we must weigh the advantages and disadvantages; our concern is that a primary focus on confirmation will prematurely restrict the range of questions asked and thereby bias the field at the outset. As Abplanalp has argued, we need to broaden our base of inquiry to address why some women believe themselves to be symptomatic even when we are unable to confirm it.[27] Of course, the strength of our argument consists in our ability to marshal convincing evidence for the benefits of clarification as opposed to confirmation.[21a]

A major impetus for making diagnoses prospectively has come from the observation that only 20 to 50 percent of retrospective, global self-reports of PMS are "confirmed" by longitudinal measures.[28,29] Table 4-1 illustrates how high and low symptom groups as assessed by global (remembered) and concurrent (actual) sources of measurement, give rise to four conceptual subgroupings.

Proponents of the biomedical model have preferred to focus on the concordant, "positive," and "negative" subgroups, neglecting the two nonconcordant cells. This preference is entirely appropriate if the discordant cells provide only "noise." How do we assess sources of variance in these subgroups if we exclude them from our studies at the outset?

TABLE 4-1. CONCORDANCE BETWEEN REMEMBERED AND ACTUAL EXPERIENCES

	Global (Remembered)	
Actual Concurrent Changes	Yes	No
Yes	Positive	False negative
No	False positive	Negative

TABLE 4-2. OVERLAPPING GROUP MEMBERSHIP

	Global (Remembered)		
Actual Concurrent Changes	Yes		No
Yes	Positive	(c)	False negative
	(a)		(b)
No	False positive		Negative

Transition from (a) positive to false positive; (b) negative to false negative; (c) false negative to positive.

INTERCHANGE BETWEEN SUBGROUPINGS AS EVIDENCE

One problem with the 2 × 2 table (Table 4-1) is that it reinforces the tendency to assume that subgroup membership is stable just because it is pictured that way. In fact, we have more reason to believe that membership in these subgroups is overlapping across time (Table 4-2). For example, a woman with seasonal variability might be confirmed as positive during the winter months but might be disproved during the summer months (false-positive (a), see Table 4-2). On the other hand, a woman who conceptualizes herself as globally negative may be confirmed as a positive (false-negative) during any given month (b); this could occur if she is beginning to have increased symptoms, as with age, but has lagged behind in self-perceptions; when she does revise them she would then become classified as positive (c). One advantage of this approach is that it encourages us to explore the interchanges between these subgroupings over time.

CYCLE REGULARITY AND SEASONAL PMS AS EVIDENCE

One source of variance in menstrual cycle symptomatology probably has to do with nonstable characteristics of cycles, e.g., regularity. Although several groups have suggested that subjects be selected on the basis of reports of regular cycles and symptoms for at least the six preceding cycles,[12] there has been little attention to the reliability of such reports. Most women in our study gave a range of several days when asked to estimate the length of their typical cycle. Ross and Vande Wiele[30] reported that only 64 percent of cycles fall into the range of past cycles when based on the ranges of the past three cycles.

These concerns are not trivial if one examines the possible relation between seasonal changes in cycles and reports of premenstrual symptoms. In a study of more than 38,000 woman-years, Sundararaj and colleagues[31] found a tendency for cycles to be longer during the winter and shorter during the summer. Although the absolute value of changes for the entire group was only a fraction of a day, we have observed women with wide variations, e.g., a 22-day cycle in the spring in contrast to a 32-day cycle in the fall. In our clinical study, 58 percent (7/12) of women who were positive for moderate to severe premenstrual symptoms in a screening interview reported seasonal changes in their menstrual symptoms, with five of them reporting exacerbations during the winter. Reciprocally, 71 percent (18/25) of women reporting seasonal affective disorder also reported premenstrual symptoms.[32]

INDIVIDUAL DIFFERENCES IN SELF-PERCEPTIONS AND RECALL AS EVIDENCE

Another source of variance may be individual differences in the acuity of self-observations[16] and thus in the remembering or reporting of symptoms. Just as women appear to be more reliable historians of psychic distress than men,[26] some women are undoubtedly more accurate than others; when overlooked, these differences may confound studies of depression in relation to the menstrual cycle. The selection of the experiences to be incorporated into long-term memory and stable self-image results from and reinforces other self-perceptions. When having been depressed is conceptualized as further evidence of one's inadequacy, it may be adaptive to selectively forget depression.

Individual differences in the selective encoding and forgetting of information about oneself premenstrually may be significant to understanding changes in reports of symptomatology over time. The so-called false-positive group during any given month probably represents, among other nontrivial processes, cognitive effects such as: (1) improvement in "positives" who benefit from the increased self-monitoring but whose global self-perception lags behind[28]; (2) changes in ratings that reflect random measurement error or responsivity to repeated testing[10]; (3) misattribution of midcycle changes to the premenstrual cycle phase, or a lag in attribution; (4) selective recall of the "worst" cycle; and (5) increased month-to-month variability in symptoms that are differentially salient to remembered self-perceptions.[21a]

Concerning the latter possibility, we examined whether symptom subscales that are the most salient to a woman's self-identified premenstrual symptoms are also the most concordant with changes in concurrent self-reports. The proportion of women in our study who globally rated themselves as high on premenstrual symptoms using the Moos questionnaire[32] and who also showed at least a 20 percent increase in symptomatology during a given cycle ranged from 17 percent (Arousal), to 29 percent (Concentration), to 71 percent (Water Retention).* The average rate of concordance across subscales in this sample was 39 percent for the globally self-identified high symptom group compared to 82 percent for the low symptom group. The frequency distributions for the concentration and pain subscales are shown in Table 4-3. A preliminary look at the data (for the Pain, Arousal, Water Retention, and Concentration subscales of the Moos questionnaire) does not show a clear relation between the salience of any retrospectively assessed symptom subscale and concordance rates with concurrent changes at the 20 percent level or greater. However, we are carefully testing this hypothesis by item and subscale correlation analysis for retrospective Moos total scores and con-

TABLE 4-3. CONCORDANCE BETWEEN REMEMBERED AND ACTUAL EXPERIENCES: GLOBAL REPORT OF OVERALL CHANGE (REMEMBERED)

Actual Changes (20%)	Concentration (%)		Pain (%)	
	Yes	No	Yes	No
Yes	29	12	58	0
No	71	88	42	100

current reports of change. An alternative hypothesis is that various symptoms are perceived or recalled with differential accuracy.

BIOLOGIC DIFFERENCES AND CORRELATES AS EVIDENCE

Finally, other evidence arguing for the study of globally defined groups (including so-called false-positives) comes from our preliminary finding that these groups differ in absolute levels of urinary 6-hydroxymelatonin across the menstrual cycle (Hamilton and Alagna, unpublished data; see also DeLisi et al[37]).[4,34] If confirmed, perhaps this biologic difference relates more to global differences in self-perceptions than to direct menstrual cycle-related effects on symptomatology during a given cycle. Similarly, we reported a trend for a globally defined group difference in urinary phenylethylamine (PEA) across the menstrual cycle, where the higher PEA levels in the high symptom group were moderately correlated with daily stress ratings.[35-37] Because of possible menstrual cycle-related effects on the neurochemical substrate of drug responsivity, we believe that more attention must be paid to the menstrual cycle as a source of variance in psychopharmacologic studies.[38,39]

CONCLUSION

Clinical investigators are urged to work toward a more human-based model for the actual conduct of research on the menstrual cycle. Proposals for selection criteria and research guidelines must be accompanied by statements about limitations in applicability. The premature use of selection criteria may restrict the range of inquiry and bias our knowledge in this field. An alternative to the overemphasis on the confirmation of premenstrual symptoms or a syndrome is the clarification of their meaning and of sources of variance in symptom expression and recollection. Just as cognition is an important variable in affective disorders research, we believe that more attention must be given to the role of altered self-perceptions in premenstrually related depressions. We have demonstrated the utility of this approach with early data from our clinical study.

ACKNOWLEDGMENT

We wish to thank Sara Pinkel, recipient of the 1984 Psychobiology of

Women Research Prize from the IRWH, who was responsible for the analysis of the data on self and observer ratings.

REFERENCES

1. McClintock MK: The behavioral endocrinology of rodents: a functional analysis. Bioscience 33:573, 1983
2. Garcia J, Koelling RA: Relation of cue to consequence in avoidance learning. Psychonom Sci 4:123, 1966
3. Ruble D: Premenstrual symptoms: a reinterpretation. Science 197:29, 1977
4. Hamilton JA, Alagna SW, Sharpe K: Cognitive approaches to understanding and treating premenstrual depressions. p. 69. In Osofsky H (ed): Premenstrual Syndromes: Current Findings and Future Directions. American Psychiatric Press, Washington, DC, 1985
5. Freedman DX: Presidential address: science in the service of the ill. Am J Psychiatry 139:1087, 1982
6. Sherif CW: Bias in psychology. In Sherman JA, Beck ET (eds): The Prism of Sex: Essays in the Sociology of Knowledge. University of Wisconsin Press, Madison, 1979
7. Unger RK: Through the looking glass: no wonderland yet! Psychol Wom Q 8:9, 1983
8. Lewontin RC, Rose S, Kamin SJ: Not in Our Genes: Biology, Ideology and Human Nature. Pantheon, New York, 1984
9. Hamilton JA, Aloi J, Mucciardi B, et al: Human plasma β-endorphin through the menstrual cycle. Psychopharmacol Bull 19:586, 1983
9a. American Psychiatric Association: p. 367. In Diagnostic and Statistical Manual, Third Edition (revised). American Psychiatric Press, Washington, DC, 1987
9b. American Medical News pp. 3, 33, 34, June 6, 1986
10. Koeske RD: Lifting the curse of menstruation: toward a feminist perspective on the menstrual cycle. Wom Health 8:1, 1983.
11. Abplanalp JM: Premenstrual syndrome: a selective review. Wom Health 8:107, 1983
12. Steiner M, Haskett RF, Carroll BJ: Premenstrual tension syndrome: the development of research diagnostic criteria and new rating scales. Acta Psychiatr Scand 62:177, 1980
13. Haskett RF, Abplanalp JM: Premenstrual tension syndrome; diagnostic criteria and selection of research subjects. Psychiatr Res 9:125, 1983
14. Rubinow DR, Roy-Byrne P, Hoban C, et al: Prospective assessment of menstrually related mood disorders. Am J Psychiatry 141:684, 1984
15. Hamilton JA, Parry BL, Alagna S, et al: Premenstrual mood changes: a guide to evaluation and treatment. Psychiatry Annu 14:426, 1984
16. Parry G, Wehr T: Research techniques used to study premenstrual syndrome. p. 85. In Osofsky H (ed): Premenstrual Syndromes: Current Findings and Future Directions. American Psychiatric Press, Washington, DC, 1985
17. Janowsky PS, Berens SC, Davis JM: Correlations between mood, weight, and electrolytes during the menstrual cycle: a renin angiotensin-aldosterone hypothesis of premenstrual tension. Psychosom Med 35:143, 1973
18. Bruce J, Russell GFM: Premenstrual tension. Lancet 2:267, 1962
19. Watson PE, Robinson MF: Variations in body-weight of young women during the menstrual cycle. Br J Nutr 19:237, 1965

20. Sommer B: How does menstruation affect cognitive competence and psychophysiological response. Wom Health 8:53, 1983

21. Alagna SW, Hamilton JA: Social stimulus perception and self-evaluation: effects of menstrual cycle phase. Psychol Wom 10:327, 1986

21a. Alagna S, Hamilton JA: Cycles of mood disorders. Paper presented at the American Psychiatric Association, Chicago, 1987 (in press)

22. Paykel ES, Prusoff BA, Klerman GL, et al: Self-report and clinical interview ratings in depression. J Nerv Ment Dis 156:166, 1973

23. Roos NP, Gaumont M, Colwell NL: Female and physician: a sex role incongruity. J Med Educ 52:345, 1977

24. Lloyd C, Gartrell NK: A further assessment of medical school stress. J Med Educ 58:964, 1983

25. Angst J, Dobler-Mikola A: Do the diagnostic criteria determine the sex ratio in depression? Paper presented at the American College of Neuropsychopharmacology, San Juan, Puerto Rico, December 1983 (abstract)

26. Mellinger GD, Balter MB, Uhlenhuth EH: Evaluating a household survey measure of psychic distress. Psychol Med 13:607, 1983

27. Abplanalp JM: The menstrual cycle: costs and benefits. Paper presented at the American Society of Psychosomatic Obstetrics and Gynecology, University of Texas Medical Branch, Galveston, 1982

28. Endicott J, Halbriech W: Retrospective reports of premenstrual changes: factors affecting confirmation by daily ratings. Psychopharmacol Bull 18:109, 1982

29. McCance RA, Luff MC, Widdowson EE: Physical and emotional periodicity in women. J Hyg (Lond) 37:571, 1937

30. Ross GT, Vande Wiele RL: The ovaries. In Williams RH (ed): Textbook of Endocrinology. p. 378. Saunders, Philadelphia, 1974

31. Sundararaj N, Chern M, Gatewood L, et al: Seasonal behavior of human menstrual cycles: a biometric investigation. Hum Biol 50:15, 1978

32. Rosenthal NE, Sack DA, Gillin JC: Seasonal affective disorder (SAD) and antidepressant effects of light. Presented at the American College of Neuropsychopharmacology, San Juan, Puerto Rico, December 1983

33. Moos RH: Menstrual Distress Questionnaire Manual. Department of Psychiatry, Stanford University, and Veterans Administration, Palo Alto, CA, 1977

34. Hamilton JA, Aloi J, Mucciardi B, et al: A neuroendocrine evaluation of premenstrual syndrome. Paper presented at the American Psychosomatic Society, New York, March 1985. Institute for Research on Women's Health, Washington DC

35. Hamilton JA, Alagna SW, Parry B, et al: An update on premenstrual depression: evaluation and treatment. In Gold J (ed): Menstrual Disorders: Implications for Clinical Psychiatry. American Psychiatric Press, Washington, DC (in press)

36. Hamilton JA, Parry B, Blumenthal S, et al: Premenstrual mood changes. Paper presented at the American Psychiatric Association, Dallas, 1985 (abstract)

37. DeLisi LE, et al: Elevated phenylethylamine in women. p. 386. In Boulton A (ed): Neuropsychopharmacology of the Trace Amines. Humana Press, Clifton, NJ, 1985

38. Hamilton JA, Conrad CD: Toward a developmental psychopharmacology: The physiological basis of age, gender, and hormonal effects on drug responsivity. p. 66. In Noshpitz JD (ed): Basic Handbook of Child Psychiatry, Vol. 5. Basic Books, New York, 1987

39. Conrad CD, Hamilton JA: Recurrent premenstrual decline in lithium concentration: Clinical correlates and treatment implications. Am J Acad Child Phychiatr 26:852, 1986

5

Evaluation of Biologic Research

Barbara L. Parry
Jeffrey L. Rausch

Late luteal phase dysphoric disorder (LLDD), the proposed term to describe disabling premenstrual symptoms, has been included in the appendix of the American Psychiatric Association's revised version of the *Diagnostic and Statistical Manual of Mental Disorders* (third edition) (*DSM-III-R*) as a "proposed diagnostic category needing further study." Critics of this diagnosis in the *DSM-III-R* argue that insufficient research in this area precludes its incorporation at this time. Whereas there has been little controversy over the existence of significant premenstrual mood changes in some women, there is yet considerable uncertainty about a precise biologic etiology of its pathogenesis. This chapter reviews the major biologic research efforts in premenstrual syndromes (PMS), addressing some of the current methodologic problems and suggesting directions for future research.

Much of what has been done in PMS research must necessarily be considered preliminary, as the size of the task requires precise tools, including accurate endocrine measurements, and diagnostic criteria, which are still under development. However, an advantage of PMS that makes it especially suitable for scientific investigation is the inherent link that exists between the premenstrual affective changes and a specific physiologic process, i.e., the menstrual cycle. In PMS both causative and curative mechanisms are entrained to the menstrual cycle. Furthermore, the mood and behavioral changes are recurrent and predictable, and therefore they can be studied both prospectively and longitudinally. The identified physiologic process of the menstrual cycle is involved in remission and relapse, and serves as a point of departure for generating hypotheses and focusing investigation into the pathogenesis of PMS.

HISTORICAL DEVELOPMENT

Menstrually related mood and behavior changes have been recognized since the time of Hippocrates. Systematic investigations into the nature and treatment of PMS, however, did not begin until the 1930s. Some of the studies were designed to test the assumption that women who reported premenstrual mood changes had higher levels of neuroticism or other forms of psychopathology as measured by psychological tests.[2-4] Frank[5] was the first to investigate a biologic hypothesis of PMS. He postulated that premenstrual symptoms resulted from excess production and decreased renal excretion of "female hormones." Since then, the development of the radioimmunoassay has allowed for the burgeoning of investigations into the role of hormones in physiology and pathophysiology. The levels of gonadal steroids can now be measured across the menstrual cycle with increasing precision and predictable patterns of secretion can be demonstrated.

BIOLOGIC HYPOTHESES OF PMS

Multiple theories have been proposed for a hormonal etiology of PMS. Each major theory is briefly reviewed, though no one theory has consistently proved to be linked to the symptoms of PMS.

GONADAL STEROIDS

Various studies have examined the possible role of gonadal hormones in the pathogenesis of PMS. Ovarian steroid theories of premenstrual mood disorder have postulated disturbances in: (1) the absolute amount of one hormone; (2) the amount of one hormone relative to that of another (estrogen–progesterone "imbalance"); (3) an idiosyncratic hormonal sensitivity; and (4) withdrawal reaction from either hormone.[6]

Frank's[5] early postulate about premenstrual symptoms was followed much later by Dalton's[7] theory that PMS is due to progesterone deficiency. However, Adamopoulos et al.[8] found no abnormal urinary excretions of total gonadotropins, estrogen, progesterones, or androgens in women with premenstrual symptoms.

Others have concluded that premenstrual symptoms of anxiety, depression, and hostility were secondary to a *relative* excess of estrogen and/or deficiency of progesterone. Israel[9] postulated that PMS was attributable to unantagonized estrogen relative to a luteal deficiency of progesterone. Endo et al.,[10] in a review of cases of periodic psychosis associated with the menstrual cycle, found frequently low urine pregnanediol levels, also suggesting a progesterone deficiency. Smith[6] focused on premenstrual depression and found mean plasma levels of progesterone during the 7 days preceding menses to be lower in rigorously defined patients with premenstrual depression compared to controls. The differences, however, though significant, were small, and estrogens were found to be normal.

Morton et al.[11] found an increase in the number of cornified cells in endometrial biopsies and smears, indicative of hyperestrogenic stimulation, in women suffering from PMS. Morton also reported inducing symptoms of premenstrual syndrome by administering intramusclar injections of estrogen.[12] In Widholm et al.'s[13] study of 514 adolescent women, those showing a hyperestrogenic pattern in vaginal smears were four to five times more likely to suffer from premenstrual tension. In contrast, Stieglitz and Kimble[14] reported normal secretory-type endometrium (implying a normal hormonal status) in 12 to 15 patients with PMS.

Cullberg[15] concluded from a study of hormonal administration that some cases of premenstrual irritability were due to estrogen dominance with a relative lack of progesterone. This theory is supported by evidence from Backstrom and Carstensen[16] who found that women with premenstrual anxiety (not well defined), compared to controls, had significantly higher plasma levels of estrogen and lower amounts of progesterone 3 to 6 days before menses. In a subsequent study, Backstrom and Mattson[17] rated symptoms of women with premenstrual syndrome into four categories of anxiety-tension, asthenia-depression, irritability-explosiveness, and feelings of swelling; they found a significant correlation between estrogen levels and anxiety and irritability ratings, which they hypothesized to be due to the excitability effect of estradiol on limbic system structures.

The studies of estrogen and progesterone in PMS in toto suggest a relative deficiency of progesterone relative to estrogen. However, there are inconsistencies with this conclusion. Though progesterone has been reported to be efficacious in treating PMS,[2,7,18] double-blind trials show progesterone to be no more efficacious than placebo.[19,20] The lack of similar mood disturbances during the preovulatory phase of the cycle, when there is a marked excess of estrogen relative to progesterone,[6] does not support mood disturbances during the premenstruum being simply a result of an increased estrogen/progesterone ratio. Because most studies of estrogen have measured estradiol, the role of the estriol/estradiol ratio may have been overlooked as a potentially significant phenomenon in causing mood disturbances.[6] Estriol has been shown to be a potent inhibitor of estradiol binding to end-organ receptor proteins.[21,22]

One modified hypothesis is that it is the level of estrogen and progesterone in relation to prolactin that affects the type of psychological symptoms reported premenstrually, but this theory requires empirical confirmation.[23] Halbreich et al.[23a] suggested that the rate of the decrease in gonadal steroids may be implicated in the pathophysiology of premenstrual mood changes.

PROLACTIN

Some, but not all, studies have shown an increase in prolactin during the luteal phase,[23-25] which might account for psychological symptoms occurring then. Halbreich et al.[26] found that women with PMS (of variable symptomatology) had higher prolactin levels throughout the cycle than nonsymptomatic women, and that the levels were increased premenstrually. Bromocriptine, a dopamine agonist that lowers the prolactin level, has been shown to alleviate premenstrual symptoms in some studies.[27-31] Though abnormally high prolactin levels are not necessarily associated with mood changes, Koppelman et al.[32] found that patients with hyperprolactinemia, compared to normal controls, reported more depressive symptoms and that the symptoms decreased when the patients were treated with bromocriptine.

We demonstrated an abnormally high prolactin level (mean 200 ng/ml) in response to thyrotropin-releasing hormone (TRH) during both midcycle and premenstrual phases in prospectively documented PMS patients; we also observed that sleep deprivation, which profoundly lowers the nighttime secretion of prolactin,[33,34] effectively alleviated symptoms in 80 percent of women with PMS documented over a 2- to 3-month interval using daily and weekly mood inventories and weekly Hamilton Rating Scales for Depression.[34a] Unlike patients with major affective disorders,[35] patients with PMS did not relapse with a night of recovery sleep but remained asymptomatic through the remainder of their premenstruum. Though further work is needed, partial or total sleep deprivation may prove to be an effective and acceptable alternative or adjunct to the pharmacologic treatment of PMS.

MINERALOCORTICOIDS

Because some premenstrual symptoms may be related to fluid retention, a mineralocorticoid hypothesis of premenstrual changes was developed implicating renin, angiotensin, and aldosterone. Janowsky et al.[36] studied 11 female college volunteers over 15 menstrual cycles, measuring daily weights, urinary potassium/sodium ratios (reflecting aldosterone effects), and self-evaluation of negative affect. They found that changes in mood were more positively correlated with changes in daily weights and urinary potassium/sodium ratios over phases of the menstrual cycle than with changes in estrogen and progesterone. They hypothesized a renin–angiotensin–aldosterone model for premenstrual syndrome: Increased progesterone levels during the luteal phase, by increasing sodium excretion, increased renin activity, which in turn activates production of angiotensin and aldosterone. Angiotensin, they speculated, may cause premenstrual symptoms by its effect on central cholinergic and possibly noradrenergic mechanisms.

A renin–angiotensin–aldosterone hypothesis of PMS is also supported by Kaulhausen et al.'s[37] report of a preovulatory and late luteal elevation of plasma renin activity that was not found in menopausal women. They suggested a strong interaction between plasma renin activity and the functional state of a woman during her menstrual cycle. This finding parallels those in other studies,[38-41] which have shown elevated levels of aldosterone during the luteal phase compared to the follicular phase of the menstrual cycle, and a doubling of angiotensin II levels during the luteal phase compared to the follicular phase of the menstrual cycle.[42] Thus progesterone/estrogen mediated changes in the renin–angiotensin–aldosterone system and might induce emotional fluctuations during different phases of the menstrual cycle.

If the PMS is related to changes in the mineralocorticoid system, one would expect diuretics, particularly aldosterone antagonists, to help alleviate the symptoms. O'Brien et al.[43] gave the aldosterone antagonist spironolactone to 28 women in a double-blind crossover trial during four menstrual cycles and reported reduced weight and relief of psychological symptoms in more than 80 percent of women in the symptomatic group. Werch and Kane[44] administered the potent diuretic metolazone (Zaroxolyn) 1 to 5 mg qd and placebo to 46 women with PMS in a double-blind crossover trial. They reported a statistically significant improvement in mood symptoms and in discomfort due to water retention. However, Mattsson and Schoultz,[45] in a study comparing lithium (24 mEq daily) to a level of 0.7 to 1.5 mEq/L, placebo, and a diuretic (chlorthalidone 25 to 50 mg qd), found that all drugs ameliorated the symptoms: placebo most, diuretics second, and lithium the least. It seems that whereas diuretics may be effective in relieving symptoms of water retention, they may be generally ineffective in treating emotional disturbances associated with PMS and are, at most, adjunctive treatment. Contrary to the mineralocorticoid hypothesis is the example of Conn's syndrome, in which aldosterone levels are elevated, and not generally associated with psychological disturbances.

PROSTAGLANDINS

Prostaglandin inhibitors are effective in treating dysmenorrhea, the cramping pain associated with the onset of menses; whether these agents might also prove effective for PMS is an open question. Some studies indicate that prostaglandins increase during the luteal phase and decline during menses.[46,47] This possibility has some physiologic basis but requires substantiation. The result of one study using mefenamic acid for treating PMS indicates a need for further study in this area,[48] utilizing PMS women without symptoms of dysmenorrhea.

ENDOGENOUS OPIATES

Because several premenstrual symptoms mimic those of narcotic withdrawal, some investigators have proposed an opiate withdrawal hypothesis of PMS.[49,50] Endorphins probably play a modulatory role in the normal menstrual cycle. Endogenous opiates inhibit luteinizing hormone (LH) release, and estrogens stimulate the hypothalamic release of β-endorphins.[51,52] In monkeys Wehrenberg et al.[53] found that cerebrospinal fluid (CSF) β-endorphins were highest during the luteal phase and were undetectable during menses. However, one plasma study of β-endorphin in humans has failed to substantiate this hypothesis.[54]

BIOGENIC AMINES

Gonadal steroids affect brain serotonin, dopamine, norepinephrine, and acetylcholine receptors and turnover.[55] These same neurotransmitters are involved, in turn, in the steroidal regulation of sexual behavior and reproductive functions. Because these neurotransmitters are thought to play a role in regulating mood and behavior in affective disorders, researchers have also explored their possible role in premenstrual affective symptomatology. Various monoamines appear to be involved in regulating the menstrual cycle. Urinary and CSF 3-methoxy-4-hydroxyphenethylene glycol (MHPG) (the central metabolite of norepinephrine), serotonin and its major metabolite 5-hydroxyindoleacetic acid (5HIAA) in urine, and monoamine oxidase have been reported to vary across the menstrual cycle in human studies.[57] A study by DeLeon-Jones et al.[58] found that women with PMS had high levels of urinary MHPG, which decreased when they were effectively treated with lithium. Parry et al. (Abstract, American College of Neuropsychopharmacology, San Juan, PR, 1983) found significantly higher levels of CSF MHPG in PMS patients during the premenstrual phase, compared to the late follicular phase. Normotensive data on monoamine changes in the normal human menstrual cycle are needed. Because the relation between gonadal steroid hormones and CNS neurotransmitters is complex, the specific nature of these reciprocal interactions and their contribution to affective changes across the menstrual cycle represents a challenge for future research.

CHRONOBIOLOGIC INVESTIGATIONS OF PMS

Chronobiologic disturbances have been implicated in the pathogenesis of major affective disorders[59] and may bear special relevance to the relation between PMS and affective disorders.[60-65] A chronobiologic hypothesis suggests that an abnormal phase relation between the oscillator controlling the sleep–wake cycle and the one controlling other circadian rhythms of rapid eye movement (REM) sleep propensity, temperature, cortisol, and melatonin may contribute to the vulnerability of individuals to develop affective illness.[59] Gonadal steroids may alter the timing of circadian rhythms and shift the activity–rest (or sleep–wake) cycle in animals.[66,67] It is conceivable that changing levels of gonadal hormones across the human menstrual cycle may disrupt normal circadian physiology in certain individuals and predispose them to the development of mood disorder during specific phases of the menstrual cycle.

Lewy et al.[68] suggested that melatonin may be used as a marker for circadian phase position. Hariharasubromanian et al.[69] examined the circadian rhythm of plasma melatonin during different phases of the normal human menstrual cycle and found a phase delay of the nocturnal peak of melatonin during midcycle. Low melatonin levels have been also reported in patients with affective illness.[70-74] We noted a delay in the onset of melatonin secretion in one patient with seasonal PMS.[74a] In this patient premenstrual symptoms occurred only during the fall and winter, in association with shortening of the daily photoperiod, and were alleviated during spring and summer in association with lengthening of the daily photoperiod. The patient was effectively treated with high-intensity light (>2,500 lux), which lowers human plasma melatonin,[75] during her symptomatic premenstrual phase. This therapeutic effect was blocked by simultaneously administering melatonin orally with the light treatment and was later reinstituted by administering propranolol and atenolol, β-antagonists, which also lower human plasma melatonin.[76,77] Beta blockers may be successful in patients with seasonal PMS, but success has yet to be determined for nonseasonal PMS. Studies are currently being conducted. Hamilton et al. (unpublished data) found a globally defined symptomatic group difference in levels of a melatonin metabolite compared to levels for a nonsymptomatic group. Cortisol measurements[69,78,79] generally do not indicate alternations of the duration or timing of secretion across the menstrual cycle.

The role of desynchronized circadian rhythms in the pathogenesis of PMS, especially if these systems are examined using experimental perturbations, may prove a promising area for future investigations.

METHODOLOGIC ISSUES

There is confusion about what constitutes normal psychological changes across the menstrual cycle. The literature frequently does not indicate what constitutes a disorder, and many studies lack delineation of criteria used to diagnose PMS. Because premenstrual symptoms may lie on a continuum from normal cyclic variations to pathologic dysfunction, it is critical to understand how patients are differentiated from controls. A prospective documentation of the nature, time, and severity of symptoms over several months is also important. At least 2 months are required for prospective ratings because 1 month is usually not representative. Attention should also be given to the evaluation process, as individual differences in self-perception, the effects of observation, and the discrepancies between subjective and objective measurements may affect the variables being measured. Furthermore, patients with PMS versus those with premenstrual exacerbations of other disorders, e.g., affective disorders or anxiety disorders, must be distinguished. As a result of a failure to address these problems, there has often been considerable heterogeneity of subject populations. This diagnostic heterogeneity may contribute to the biologic heterogeneity found in PMS patients and may make it difficult to compare the findings of the various studies.

The method by which hypotheses have been developed in PMS research warrants review. From an examination of patterns of evaluation between specified variables in PMS research to date (i.e., hormone levels and mood, or menstrual cycle phase and mood state), one cannot infer a clear causal relation. The strategies employed provide useful descriptions of the syndromes, but the hypotheses generated from this approach need to be systematically investigated using pharmacologic or other experimental manipulations. Many neuroregulatory processes may vary across the menstrual cycle but may not be involved in PMS.

Furthermore, the inference of causes of PMS from treatment responses is a limited strategy. Effective treatment may act through a mechanism independent of the one responsible for PMS. Another pitfall of inferring pathogenesis from treatment response is the high rate of placebo response (about 60 percent) in PMS.[80]

There are several problems with the approach of measuring hormone levels as a strategy to determine the etiology of PMS. Marked intra- and interindividual variability occur in gonadal steroid hormone secretion across the normal menstrual cycle, making it difficult to determine the degree of fluctuation that indicates pathology. Many investigators of PMS have interpreted changes in such variables as abnormal, short of defining normal menstrual cycle variation.

Another methodologic problem in PMS research is the variance in the timing of measurements. In subjects with different cycle lengths, the same cycle day may reflect different menstrual cycle phases. Reliance on external time markers, rather than internal ones, e.g., cytologic, hormonal, or body temperature measurements, can cause increased variability due to menstrual phase differences and contribute to the inconsistency of findings. Also, in order to determine changes associated with an approximate 28-day cycle, spans between successive measurements should be short enough, i.e., no more than 7 days, in order to discern a pattern. Many studies have used single time points to determine measurements. This approach does not take into account circadian and monthly rhythmic variations and does not lend itself to understanding how biologic processes change over time. The timing of measurements with regard to the month of the year should be reported as there may be circannual changes in menstrual rhythms.[81]

Thus although much investigation has been done into the nature and treatment of PMS, some methodologic problems in these studies have limited their usefulness. Studies in the future that address these methodologic issues and that are designed to test specific hypotheses using experimental perturbations will help focus, and thereby enhance, the quality of research in PMS.

FUTURE DIRECTIONS

Probably the single most rate-limiting factor in PMS research is diagnosis. Clinicians and investigators need standardized diagnostic criteria that delineate the type of symptoms, their severity, and their timing with respect to the menstrual cycle. Whether there are specific subtypes of PMS also requires further validation.

The relation of PMS to affective disorders needs to be more fully addressed. Some, but not all, studies indicate that a high percentage of PMS patients either have a history of or later develop an affective disorder.[60-65,82,83] It is not clear whether having PMS constitutes a risk for affective illness or other reproductive-related affective disturbances, such as those that occur with oral contraceptives, during pregnancy and the puerperium, and at menopause. Such questions require prospective, longitudinal investigation. It is possible, for example, that an episode of affective illness linked to the reproductive cycle sensitizes a woman to the development of subsequent depressions or affects the rate of recurrence of future affective illness. Using sound methodology, the investigation of endocrine, monoamine, and chronobiologic associations in patients with carefully documented affective symptoms may shed light on this perplexing interface of biology and psychology.

In summary, the achievement of sound biologic research in PMS requires an examination of the perception of premenstrual symptoms, delineating specific diagnostic criteria and documenting clinical, psychosocial, and biologic characteristics of identified subgroups of patients. Toward this goal we have reviewed the reported studies, examining certain methodologic problems that limit their usefulness and identifying specific areas of investigation which in future studies would facilitate progress in PMS research.

REFERENCES

1. American Psychiatric Association: Diagnostic and Statistical Manual of Mental Disorders, Third Edition, Revised. American Psychiatric Association, Washington, DC, 1987
2. Rees C: The premenstrual tension syndrome and its treatment. Br Med J 1:1014, 1953
3. Paulson MJ: Psychological concomitants of premenstrual tension. Am J Obstet Gynecol 81:733, 1961
4. Novell HA: Psychological factors in premenstrual tension and dysmenorrhea. Clin Obstet Gynecol 8:222, 1965
5. Frank RT: The hormonal causes of premenstrual tension. Arch Neurol Psychiatry 26:1053, 1931
6. Smith SL: Mood and the menstrual cycle. p. 19. In Sachar EJ (ed): Topics in Psychoendocrinology. Grune & Stratton, Orlando, FL, 1975
7. Dalton K: The Premenstrual Syndrome and Progesterone Therapy. Heinemann, London, 1977
8. Adamopoulos DA, Loraine JA, Lunn SF, et al: Endocrine profiles in premenstrual tension. Clin Endocrinol (Oxf) 1:283, 1972
9. Israel SL: Premenstrual tension. JAMA 110:1721, 1941
10. Endo M, Darguji M, Asano Y, et al: Periodic psychosis recurring in association with menstrual cycle. J Clin Psychiatry 39:456, 1978
11. Morton JH, Addison H, Addison RG, et al: A clinical study of premenstrual tension. Am J Obstet Gynecol 65:1182, 1953
12. Morton JH: Premenstrual tension. Am J Obstet Gynecol 60:343, 1950
13. Widholm O, Frisk M, Tenhunen T, Hortling H: Gynecological findings in adolescence. Acta Obstet Gynecol Scand [Suppl 1] 46:1, 1967
14. Stieglitz EJ, Kimble ST: Premenstrual intoxication. Am J Med Sci 218:616, 1949
15. Cullberg J: Mood changes and menstrual symptoms with different gestagen/estrogen combinations. Acta Psychiatr Scand [Suppl] 236:1, 1972
16. Backstrom T, Cartensen H: Estrogen and progesterone in plasma in relation to premenstrual tension. J Biochem 5:257, 1974
17. Backstrom T, Mattson B: Correlation in symptoms in premenstrual tension to estrogen and progesterone concentrations in blood plasma. Neuropsychobiology 1:80, 1975
18. Gray LA: The use of progesterone in nervous tension states. South Med J 34:1004, 1941
19. Jordheim O: The premenstrual syndrome. Acta Ostet Gynecol Scand 51:77, 1972
20. Sampson GA: Premenstrual syndrome: a double-blind controlled trial of progesterone and placebo. Br J Psychiatry 135:209, 1979
21. Wotiz HH, Scublinsky A: The contraceptive action of impending estrogens. II. Post coital effects of estriol in the rat. J Reprod Fertil 26:143, 1971
22. Brecher PI, Wotiz HH: Competition between estradiol and estriol for end organ receptor proteins. Steroids 9:431, 1967

23. Carroll BJ, Steiner M: The psychobiology of premenstrual dysphoria: the role of prolactin. Psychoneuroendocrinology 3:171, 1978

23a. Halbreich U, Endicott J, Goldstein S, Nee J: Premenstrual changes and changes in gonadal hormones. Acta Psychother Scand 74:576, 1986

24. Franchimont P, Dourcy C, LeGross JJ, et al: Prolactin levels during the menstrual cycle. Clin Endocrinol (Oxf) 5:643, 1976

25. Vekemans M, Deluoye P, L'Iternite M: Serum prolactin levels during the menstrual cycle. J Clin Endocrinol Metab 44:989, 1977

26. Halbreich U, Ben-David M, Assail M, et al: Serum-prolactin in women with premenstrual syndrome. Lancet 1:654, 1976

27. Benedek-Jaszmann LJ, Hearn-Sturtevant MD: Premenstrual tension and functional infertility. Lancet 1:1095, 1976

28. Andersch B, Hahn L, Wendersterm C, Abrahamsen L: Treatment of the premenstrual tension syndrome with bromocriptine. Acta Endocrinol [Suppl 216] (Copenh) 88:165, 1978

29. Andersen AN, Larsen JF, Stienstrup OR, et al: Effect of bromocriptine on the premenstrual syndrome: a double-blind clinical trial. Br J Obstet Gynaecol 84:370, 1977

30. Andersen AN, Larsen JF: Bromocriptine in the treatment of the premenstrual syndrome. Drugs 17:383, 1979

31. Ghose K, Coppen A: Dromocriptine and premenstrual syndrome: controlled study. Br Med J 15:147, 1977

32. Koppelman MCS, Parry BL, Hamilton JA, et al: Libido and affect in hyperprolactinemia: Effect of biamacriptine on a randomized double-blinded placebo crossover. Am J Psychiatry (in press)

33. Sassin JF, Frantz AG, Kapen S, et al: The nocturnal rise of human prolactin is dependent on sleep. J Clin Endocrinol Metab 37:436, 1973

34. Parker DC, Rossman LG, Vanderlaan EF: Sleep related, nyctohemeral and briefly episodic variation in human plasma prolactin concentrations. J Clin Endocrinol Metab 36:1119, 1973

34a. Hamilton M: Development of a rating scale for primary depressive illness. Br J Soc Clin Psychol 6:278, 1967

35. Gillin JC: The sleep therapies of depression. Prog Neuropsychopharmacol Biol 7:351, 1983

36. Janowsky DS, Berens SC, David JM: Correlations between mood, weight, electrolyes during the menstrual cycle: a renin-angiotensin-aldosterone hypothesis of premenstrual tension. Psychosom Med 35:143, 1973

37. Kaulhausen H, Oehm W, Breuer H: Plasma renin activity during the normal menstrual cycle. Acta Endocrinol [Suppl] (Copenh) 173:160, 1973

38. Gray MJ, Strausfeld RS, Wantanabe M: Aldosterone secretory rates in the normal menstrual cycle. J Clin Endocrinol Metab 28:1269, 1968

39. Reich M: The variations in urinary aldosterone values of normal females during the menstrual cycle. Aust Ann Med 11:41, 1962

40. Katz FH, Roman P: Plasma aldosterone and renin activity during the menstrual cycle. J Clin Endocrinol 34:819, 1972

41. Schwartz VD, Abraham GE: Corticosteroid and aldosterone levels during the menstrual cycle. Obstet Gynecol 45:339, 1975

42. Sundsfjord JA, Aakvaag A: Plasma angiotension II and aldosterone excretion during the menstrual cycle. Acta Endocrinol (Copenh) 64:432, 1970

43. O'Brien PMS, Craven D, Selby C, Symonds EM: Treatment of premenstrual syndrome by spironolactone. Br J Obstet Gynaecol 86:142, 1979

44. Werch A, Kane RE: Treatment of premenstrual tension with metolazone: a double-blind evaluation of a new diuretic. Curr Ther Res 19:565, 1976
45. Mattsson B, Schoultz B: A comparison between lithium, placebo, and a diuretic in premenstrual tension. Acta Psychiatr Scand [Suppl] 225:75, 1974
46. Pulkkinen MO, Csapo AI: Effect of ibuprofen on menstrual blood prostaglandin levels in dysmenorrheic women. Prostaglandins 18:137, 1979
47. Koullapis EN, Collins WP: The concentration of 13,14-dehydro-15-oxoprostaglandin F_2 in a peripheral venous plasma throughout the normal ovarian and menstrual cycle. Acta Endocrinol (Copenh) 93:123, 1980
48. Wood C, Jacubowicz D: The treatment of premenstrual symptoms with mefenamic acid. Br J Obstet Gynaecol 87:627, 1980
49. Reid RL, Yen SSC: Premenstrual syndrome. Am J Obstet Gynecol 139:85, 1981
50. Halbriech U, Endicott J: Possible involvement of endorphin withdrawal or imbalance in specific premenstrual syndromes and postpartum depression. Med Hypothesis 7:1045, 1981
51. Quigley MH, Yen SSC: The role of endogenous opiates on LH secretion during the menstrual cycle. J Clin Endocrinol Metab 51:179, 1980
52. Ferin M: Endogenous opioid peptides and the menstrual cycle. Trends Neurosci 194:June, 1984
53. Wehrenberg WB, Wardlow SL, Frantz AG, et al: β-Endorphin in hypophyseal portal blood: variations throughout the menstrual cycle. Endocrinology 111:879, 1982
54. Hamilton JA, Aloi J, Mucciardi B, et al: Human plasma beta-endorphin throughout the menstrual cycle. Psychopharmacol Bull 19:586, 1983
55. McEwen BS, Parsons B: Gonadal steroid action on the brain: neurochemistry and neuropharmacology. Annu Rev Pharmacol Toxicol 22:555, 1982
56. Bandano AR, Nagle CA, Casas PRF, et al: Plasma levels of norepinephrine during the periovulatory period in normal women. Am J Obstet Gynecol 131:299, 1978
57. Rausch JL, Janowsky DS: Premenstrual tension: etiology. p. 397. In Friedman RC (ed): Behavior and the Menstrual Cycle. Marcel Dekker, New York, 1982
58. DeLeon-Jones FA, Val E, Herts C: MHPG excretion and lithium treatment during premenstrual tension syndrome. Am J Psychiatry 139:950, 1982
59. Wehr TA: Biological rhythms and manic depressive illness. p. 190. In Post RM, Ballenger JC (eds): Neurobiology of Mood Disorders. Williams & Wilkins, Baltimore, 1984
60. Endicott J, Halbreich U, Schacht S, Nee J: Premenstrual changes and affective disorders. Psychosom Med 43:519, 1981
61. Halbreich U, Endicott J: Relationship of dysphoric premenstrual changes to depressive disorders. Acta Psychiatr Scand 71:331, 1985
62. Hallman J: The premenstrual syndrome—an equivalent of depression? Acta Psychatr Scand 73:403, 1986
63. MacKenzie TB, Wilcox K, Baron H: Lifetime prevalence of psychiatric disorders in women with premenstrual difficulties. J Affective Disord 10:15, 1986
64. Schuckit MA, Daly V, Herman G, et al: Premenstrual symptoms and depression in a university population. Dis Nerv Sys 36:516, 1975
65. Wetzel RD, Reich T, McClure JN, et al: Premenstrual affective syndrome and affective disorder. Br J psychiatry 127:129, 1975
66. Morin LP, Fitzgerald KM, Zucker I: Estradial shortens the period of hamster circadian rhythms. Science 196:305, 1977
67. Albers HE, Gerall AA, Axelson JF: Effect of reproductive state on circadian periodicity in the rat. Physiol Behav 26:21, 1981
68. Lewy AJ, Sack RC, Single CM: Assessment and treatment of chronobiologic disor-

ders using plasma melatonin levels and bright light exposure: the clock gate model and the phase response curve. Psychopharmacol Bull 20:561, 1984

69. Hariharasubromanian N, Nair NPV, Pilapil C: Circadian rhythm of plasma melatonin and sortisol during the menstrual cycle. In Brown GM, Wainwright SD (eds): The Pineal Gland: Endocrine Aspects. Pergamon Press, Oxford, 1984

70. Wetterberg L, Beck-Friis J, Aperia B, Petterson U: Melatonin/cortisol ratio in depression. Lancet 2:1361, 1979

71. Mendlewicz J, Branchey L, Weinberg U, et al: The 24-hour pattern of plasma melatonin in depressed patients before and after treatment. Commun Psychopharmacol 4:49, 1980

72. Wirz-Justice A, Arendt J: Diurnal, menstrual cycle, and seasonal indole rhythms in man and their modification in affective disorders. p. 294. In Obiols J, Baiws C, Moncluse G, Pujol J (eds): Biological Psychiatry Today. Elsevier/North Holland, Amsterdam, 1979

73. Brown R, Kocsis JH, Caroff S, et al: Differences in nocturnal melatonin secretion between melancholic depressed patients and controls. Am J Psychiatry 142:811, 1985

74. Claustrat B, Chazot G, Brun J, et al: A chronobiological study of melatonin and cortisol secretion in depressed subjects: plasma melatonin, a biochemical marker in major depression. Biol Psychiatry 19:1215, 1984

74a. Parry BL, Rosenthal NE, Tamarkin L, Webr TA: Treatment of a patient with seasonal premenstrual syndrome. Am J Psychiatry 144:762, 1987

75. Lewy AJ, Wehr TA, Goodwin FK, et al: Light suppresses melatonin secretion in humans. Science 210:1267, 1980

76. Hanssen T, Hedyder T, Sunberg I, Wetterberg L: Effect of propranolol on serum melatonin. Lancet 2:309, 1977

77. Cowen PJ, Fraser S, Sammous R, Green AR: Atenolol reduces plasma melatonin concentration in man. Br J Clin Pharmacol 15:579, 1983

78. Haskett RF, Steiner M, Carroll BJ: A psychoendocrine study of premenstrual tension syndrome. J Affective Disord 6:191, 1984

79. Steiner M, Haskett RF, Carroll BJ: Circadian hormone secretory profiles in women with severe premenstrual tension syndrome. Br J Obstet Gynaecol 91:466, 1984

80. Day JB: Clinical trials in premenstrual syndrome. Curr Med Res Opin 6:suppl. 5, 40, 1979

81. Reinberg A, Smolensky H: Circatrigintan secondary rhythms related to hormonal changes in the menstrual cycle: general considerations. In Ferin M, Halberg F, Richard R, et al (eds): Biorhythms and Human Reproduction. Wiley, New York, 1974

82. Diamond SB, Rubinstein AA, Dunner DL, et al: Menstrual problems in women with primary affective illness. Compr Psychiatry 17:541, 1976

83. Haskett RF, Steiner M, Osmun JN, et al: Severe premenstrual tension: delineation of the syndrome. Biol Psychiatry 15:1, 1980

6

Gynecologic PMS Program: Hormonal Influences on Symptom Manifestation

Steven J. Sondheimer
Ellen Freeman
Karl Rickels

Reproductive-age women have hormonal fluctuations that are a normal part of the ovulatory cycle. Pituitary follicle-stimulating hormone (FSH), luteinizing hormone (LH), ovarian estrogen, and progesterone vary. Hypothalamic gonadotropin-releasing hormone (GnRH) is released in a pulsatile fashion that does not need to vary during the cycle for ovulation to occur, but in women pulse frequency probably does decrease during the luteal phase.[1] Androgens, adrenal hormones, and possibly central neurotransmitters vary to some degree during the cycle.

The relation between these known physiologic events and the symptomatology popularly known as premenstrual syndrome (PMS) continues to be elusive. Most women are aware of physical changes in relation to the menstrual cycles, and some 10 to 20 percent report symptoms, either physical or emotional, that are severe to disabling.[2] Whether a premenstrual syndrome applies to the latter group is the focus of current research.

WHAT IS PMS?

PMS refers to a constellation of somatic and affective changes that have a cyclicity related to the menstrual cycle.[3] Symptoms occur during the luteal phase of the menstrual cycle and abate following menstruation. Diagnosing PMS includes confirming the following conditions

1. Cyclicity of symptoms with relation to menses
2. Symptom distress occurring premenstrually

3. Symptom abatement or remission following menses

4. Premenstrual symptoms resulting in moderate to severe impairment of functioning

5. Symptoms that are recurrent for at least 6 months

6. Symptoms that are prospectively reported for at least two of three menstrual cycles

Although more than 150 symptoms have been linked with PMS, the predominant symptoms agreed on include the affective symptoms of depressed mood, anxiety, feelings of irritability, a sense of loss of control, and erratic mood changes; somatic symptoms include bloatedness, breast tenderness, abdominal discomfort and pain, headaches, and fatigue.[4]

DIAGNOSIS AND CLASSIFICATION

Classifying patients who present with premenstrual symptoms presents a challenge to the clinician. In our program patient classification is based on the daily symptoms reporting logs completed by the patient and several psychological assessments performed by a trained counselor post- and premenstrually.

DAILY SYMPTOM REPORT

The most useful diagnostic tool for the medical practitioner is a prospective daily symptom report maintained by the patient for at least three menstrual cycles before hormonal or psychotropic medications are prescribed. This self-assessment identifies the specific symptoms, the days they occur in relation to menses, and the intensity of each symptom rated on a 0- to 4-point scale. It is important that the patient maintain this record on a daily basis, as retrospective reports of the timing and intensity of symptoms have been shown to be unreliable and to overdiagnose PMS.[5]

Any existing symptom patterns should emerge from the patient's series of reports. More than one cycle report is needed because of the large variation between individual cycles and because symptoms may change following the diagnostic evaluation.[6] If symptoms occur throughout the cycle, a significant increase in intensity or the emergence of other, additional symptoms should be observed during the premenstruum. Symptoms that occur randomly throughout the cycle or do not have a cyclic relation with menses are not symptoms of a premenstrual syndrome. It is important to emphasize that it is unlikely that a patient's symptom report will be identical each month, and that identical reports suggest invalid recording, as individual variations in the timing and intensity of symptoms are usual.

A broad definition of PMS is that symptoms on days 22 to 28 (of a standardized 28-day cycle) are significantly higher than symptoms on days 6 to 12, as evidenced over two or three cycles of prospective daily symptom reports preceding treatment.[7] Patients who meet these criteria can be further classified into subgroups according to severity of postmenstrual symptoms and degree of premenstrual increase reported on the daily symptom records.[8]

We have classified PMS patients into three groups based on objective criteria applied to the pretreatment daily symptom reports.

PMS: few or no symptoms following menses with a more than 50 percent increase in premenstrual symptoms. A *significant* change is essential. The National Institute of Mental Health (NIMH) guidelines call for at least a 30 percent change.

Possible PMS: moderate postmenstrual symptoms with a more than 50 percent increase in premenstrual symptoms. Also called menstrual distress syndrome (MDS). It is characterized by symptoms throughout the period that worsen premenstrually and is associated with a coexistent psychiatric diagnosis. The patient is without a symptom-free period.

No PMS: moderate to severe postmenstrual symptoms with less than a 50 percent increase in premenstrual symptoms.

Though a classification system based on symptom clusters was an early attempt by Abraham to bring order, we have not found in our patients that these clusters are independent, and we do not use it.[9,10] This group may include mild PMS, probably a different entity from severe PMS.

PSYCHOLOGICAL ASSESSMENT

DIAGNOSTIC INTERVIEW

In addition to the daily symptom record, we have utilized an array of psychological instruments as part of a standardized diagnostic interview. The primary instruments include the Hamilton Rating Scales of Depression[11] and Anxiety[12] and the Depression portion of the Schedule for Affective Disorders and Schizophrenia (SADS).[13] By using these instruments, the clinician determines if a patient meets the accepted criteria for Affective Disorder as classified in the *Diagnostic and Statistical Manual of the American Psychiatric Association (DSM-III)*.[11,12]

We have found such diagnosis to be of interest in the further classification of our patient population. For example, the No PMS and Possible PMS groups have a strong association with current psychiatric illness including major depression and generalized anxiety disorder, whereas less than 20 percent of the women in the PMS group meet *DSM-III* criteria for major affective disorder.[8]

The question of treating a coexisting psychiatric disorder is problematic. It has been our practice to refer for psychiatric treatment patients who meet the diagnostic criteria for major depressive disorder no matter to which PMS diagnostic criteria group they are assigned. However, the patients meeting the criteria for other nonpsychotic affective disorders are included in the PMS study population to be evaluated in a double-blind controlled treatment outcome study to determine possible relations between diagnostic classification and treatment response.

MMPI SCALES

The Minnesota Multiphasic Personality Inventory (MMPI),[14,15] a widely used measure of behavioral and emotional disorders, further delineates two groups of the PMS population. The MMPI is administered during the postmenstrual (follicular) phase of the cycle. MMPI standard scores on the clinical scales are well within the normal range in the PMS group, whereas scores are significantly higher ($p < 0.01$) on 6 of 10 scales in the Possible PMS and No PMS groups.[8] Thirty-five percent of the PMS group have elevated scores (i.e., one or more clinical scores of more than 70) compared to 82 percent in the combined Possible PMS and No PMS groups.[8]

The MMPI profile of the PMS group suggests the presence of moderate tension, anxiety, headaches, and difficulties in close relationships. Such patients profit from support and reassurance and have a good response to psychotherapy.[15] The MMPI profile of the Possible PMS and No PMS groups (which do not differ statistically) suggests the presence of depression, nervousness, no clear-cut physical symptoms, and long histories of vague complaints. Such patients report fatigue and exhaustion and are often preoccupied with personal deficiencies and problematic relationships. They characteristically have little insight, poor hostility control, and poor treatment response.[15]

HORMONAL INFLUENCES ON SYMPTOM MANIFESTATION

The current level of understanding of hormonal influence on premenstrual affective symptoms remains limited.[16] Nonetheless, there are a number of theories that have been projected based on the known effects of gonadal steroids. Although more research is required to ascertain their validity, these theoretical possibilities can be informative in setting the direction for further research.

GONADAL STEROIDS

Most patients with PMS have normal luteal function. Most (but not all) studies have not been able to show a clear progesterone deficiency during the luteal phase in premenstrual syndrome patients.[17,18]

Although an older study by Backstrom et al. showed a decrease progesterone level or an increased estrogen/progesterone ratio during the second half of the cycle in PMS patients, these authors were subsequently not able to replicate their finding.[19] Furthermore, the negative affective states are often well established before the progesterone decrease begins. If there were a progesterone deficiency during the luteal phase, we would have expected to find an increased incidence of infertility, which we have not, in more than 600 patients seeking treatment in our PMS program. We know too that exercise, sleep deprivation, and other stressors may decrease luteal phase progesterone. Therefore lower progesterone, when present, may be an effect rather than a cause.[20] Certainly, there is no evidence that serum levels of gonadal hormones—estrogen and progesterone—are at all useful in diagnosing individual patients with PMS.[21]

Gonadal hormones may mediate mood changes by their effects on central neurotransmitters. Unfortunately, there is as yet no good measure to look at central nervous system sensitivity. There have been a number of theories based on known effects of gonadal steroids. However, at this point there is no evidence that these theories are valid even though they make theoretical sense. For example, monoamine oxidase (MAO), one of the major catabolic enzymes of the biogenic amines, can be measured in plasma (though not necessarily reflecting central activity). Plasma MAO activity varies with the menstrual cycle. It is low just before ovulation and high during the premenstrual phase of the cycle. There is additional evidence to suggest that estrogen can elevate mood by inhibiting MAO activity and enhancing central norepinephrine production. During the second half of the cycle MAO activity is not inhibited and could be responsible for decreased mood, depression, or inhibition of manic activity.[22] Experimental animal data support the reports that gonadal steroids have an effect on behavior.[23] There is also indirect evidence that estrogen and progesterone affect the human brain; for example, there is normal variation in the electroencephalogram (EEG) during the cycle.[24]

Another popular theory on affective symptoms during the menstrual cycle revolves around endogenous opiate peptides (EOPs) or endorphins.[25,26] Oophorectomy decreases hypothalamic EOP activity, whereas replacement of gonadal steroids (estrogen and progesterone) causes an increase in this activity. There is also human evidence that hypothalamic opiate activity is increased during the midluteal phase when estrogen and progesterone are elevated. This theory then goes on to suggest that increased endogenous opiate activity may lead to fatigue and depression, and as gonadal steroids decrease there may be precipitation of irritability, anxiety, and tension, as seen during narcotic withdrawal. Though an occasional patient's behavioral complaints seem to be consistent with this hypotheses (i.e., some increase in symptoms as the estrogen level falls after the midcycle surge with the return of symptoms with the fall in estrogen and progesterone) in general, most patients' complaints cannot be so easily related to this type of cyclic fluctuation. Though the opiate activity and withdrawal theory is attractive, and though both hypothalamic and peripheral opiate activity vary with the menstrual cycle, there is still little evidence that this change is actually the *cause* of women's symptomatology.

Similarly, 5-hydroxyindoleacetic acid (5-HIAA), a metabolite of serotonin, is known to be higher during the luteal phase than during the follicular phase and to decrease concomitantly with progesterone withdrawal,[27] but the association of these changes is no proof of a causal relation.

In another example, estrogens enhance liver conversion of the serotonin precursor tryptophan to nicotinic acid, thus possibly decreasing the tryptophan available to produce serotonin in the brain. This mechanism may play a part in the depression seen in women on birth control pills.[28] Cyclic variations do occur, and we should expect women to perceive different parts of the cycle differently. However, which if any of these changes are the keys to premenstrual syndrome is unclear.

It is likely that the same neurotransmitters thought to moderate affective disorders are operative in premenstrual affective changes as well. A complex model might be devised where the patient's neuropsychiatric state, i.e., underlying concomitant psychological state, is affected and moderated by environmental and stress-related changes in neurotransmitters. Changes in gonadal steroids change neurotransmitter levels. This last step potentially has two parts. First, gonadal steroids direct effects centrally. Secondly, the gonadal steroid effect on cardiac output, fluid status, or other somatic changes then signal, via a psychological or learned response, the central effects.

RECOGNITION OF OTHER SYSTEMIC DISORDERS

An important caveat for the clinician presented with the patient with the apparent symptoms of PMS is the importance of remaining alert to systemic diseases that are also often present with a variety of somatic and affective symptoms that vary in intensity over time. Although routine hormone screening of PMS patients is not useful, it is important for the clinician to remain alert to the possibility of hyperparathyroidism, diabetes, collagen vascular disease, and thyroid or adrenal disease.

Hyperparathyroidism (more common in women) in its earliest stages, in addition to causing diffuse aches and pains, may produce muscle weakness, anorexia, nausea, and constipation. The increased calcium may be associated with polyuria and polydipsia. Behavioral changes can be seen as well.

Behavioral changes may be present as the earliest manifestation of a collagen vascular disease such as lupus or an endocrine abnormality such as hyperthyroidism. Abdominal cramping with behavioral changes may be part of porphyria as well as diabetes or a collagen vascular disease. Though cyclic abdominal pain has been reported in some patients with acute intermittent porphyria, most do not have cyclic variation. However, in some illnesses a woman might perceive that her symptoms are cyclic. Therefore a complete medical "review of symptoms" as well as a review of the prospective "calendars" is necessary. With this information, selective screening can be undertaken using a blood calcium level, thyroid function tests, the Watson-Schwartz test for porphyria, or screening tests for collagen vascular disease such the antinuclear antibody test or erythrocyte sedimentation rate.

The patient who has a completely negative review of symptoms, regular ovulatory cycles, a normal physical examination, and a symptom calendar showing premenstrual affective or physical symptoms does not need routine blood tests. This view from a gynecologic perspective may not be shared by internists, who consider blood work routine, or by psychiatrists, who are concerned about missing physical illness.

WATER RETENTION

One of the well documented normal premenstrual changes is a feeling of water retention, though there is not necessarily actual weight gain or increase in girth.[20,30] It has been long suggested that PMS might be related to hormones that are responsible for fluid balance. Although individual patients have been seen who have marked fluctuations during the cycle, there is no study that shows a relation between weight change and other symptoms during the premenstruum.

Why then do some patients have breast tenderness, food cravings, and bloating? The normal hormonal shifts might cause changes that explain each of these symptoms. For example, progesterone during the luteal phase causes insulin resistance as measured by decreased insulin receptors on monocytes. However, individual glucose tolerance tests have not yet been shown to identify these patients.[31] Complex interactions of socialization and psychological makeup probably bring out this tendency. Individual variations in organs such as the breast might make individuals more susceptible to changes in fluids, estrogen, or prolactin.

NORMAL PREMENSTRUAL EVENTS

Lahmeyer et al.[29] reported on a group of 11 normal women, mostly in their twenties, who were followed in detail during a cycle. All of these women had intensive selection interviews, including baseline psychological tests and family histories, and were chosen from a larger group of women who had agreed to participate in the study. These women appeared to be psychologically normal and did not complain of PMS per se. They were followed without knowing the nature of the study and so were treated anytime during the cycle. None of the premenstrual affective symptoms evaluated had a significant premenstrual increase. For example, anxiety, as measured by the Spielberger State Anxiety Scale, showed a trend to premenstrual increase, but it did not reach statistical significance because of the large deviation across the cycle. The only symptom to reach statistical significance premenstrually was a feeling of water retention, although actual weight gain was not documented.

Others have also documented that there is a premenstrual increase in feeling of water retention but not an actual increase in abdominal girth or weight.[30] Because so many women note that their clothes, especially the tighter-fitting clothes, are even tighter premenstrually, perhaps these tight-fitting clothes are a more sensitive indicator of fluid shifts than standard measures of abdominal girth.

The feeling of bloatedness premenstrually may be due to a redistribution of body fluid into the abdomen or into the wall of the gut. However, it may also be due to gaseous distention of the large bowel secondary to the smooth muscle relaxing effect of progesterone during the luteal phase.[32]

In normal ovulating women, then, there is often a premenstrual change in body perception, mainly this awareness of water retention or bloating. There also may be a tendency toward increased anxiety in normal women without complaints of premenstrual symptoms, but in most individuals there are such daily fluctuations due to life events that it is difficult to document a premenstrual increase.

The temporal relation between gonadal hormonal changes and the feelings of water retention and bloatedness suggest a causal link but do not prove it. Though patients with PMS may, in general, perceive their water retention and bloatedness as being worse, they do not necessarily have a documented increase in weight. Furthermore, though weight changes do occur in some women premenstrually and though some of these women complain of affective symptoms as well, when these conditions are followed prospectively it appears that there is no clear relation between weight change and affective symptoms. Weight changes have not been related to the severity of the other premenstrual symptoms.

It is possible that certain women, because of their psychological makeup, overreact to somatic changes in their bodies. However, it is also possible that hormonal changes that normally cause a shift in fluid distribution or gastrointestinal motility cause other central hormonal changes to which some women, for psychological, environmental, or genetic reasons, are more susceptible.

Another possibility is that certain women, similar to women with dysmenorrhea, may have more extreme levels of cyclic hormones or respond chemically to a greater degree to normal hormonal changes. However, at this point, few data are available, perhaps because the elusive changes are occurring centrally and are not reflected in plasma levels. Furthermore, it is likely that different premenstrual symptoms have different explanations.

TREATMENT

NONSPECIFIC SUPPORTIVE THERAPY

There is accumulating evidence that in the absence of any known etiology of PMS the most appropriate initial treatment is supportive, educational counseling in the areas of nutrition, exercise, stress management, and the patient's self-awareness about her specific symptom constellation.

We have found that the process of identifying and learning to understand the symptoms and their patterns is itself therapeutic. Prospective daily symptom reporting and diagnostic interviews help patients learn that their symptoms are not unpredictable and overwhelming but occur at a specific time and can be managed. Group discussions help women perceive that their experiences are not isolated or even highly unusual.[33] These discussions encourage them to learn different behavior patterns and coping mechanisms that can reduce symptoms.

The diagnostic interview process can be of particular therapeutic value through discussion of the prospective symptom chart and of specific symptom patterns, and the teaching of certain coping strategies.

Good nutrition and exercise—hallmarks of good health—can also decrease premenstrual symptoms. Reducing salt intake (particularly if symptoms of edema are present), eliminating caffeine, nicotine, alcohol, and recreational and/or abused drugs, reducing sugar intake, and regularly eating small, well-balanced meals result in some improvement for most women who seek medical treatment for PMS. Exercise can improve muscle tone, relieve aches, and reduce tension and irritability. Exercise may also alter central neurotransmitters.

It is unlikely that dietary inadequacy is actually the cause of premenstrual changes or that dietary changes "cure" PMS. Rather, the patient who is sensitive to hormonal fluctuations—body awareness—is also sensitive to the stimulative effects of caffeine, the catecholamine rush of free sugars, or the effects of alcohol. Furthermore, feeling good about oneself from exercise improves the response to body changes. These nonmedicated approaches should be implemented before hormonal therapy.

Our PMS treatment program includes an intensive review of nutrition and exercise, participation in a group session, maintenance of daily symptom reports for one or two cycles, and prescription of 200 mg of vitamin B_6 and a multivitamin daily.

In this group of patients approximately one-third reported global responses of "good" improvement after two cycles of these initial treatments. However, after 6 months, only 17 percent continued the initial regimen and maintained good improvement.[34] This figure suggests that many initial responders experienced only short-term relief. Whether improvement in the initial treatment regimen results from vitamin B_6 cannot be determined without well-designed double-blind, crossover, placebo-controlled studies. It is of interest that the 17 percent persistent "good" responders to conservative treatment were the patients with the fewest postmenstrual affective symptoms.[34]

A large placebo response is identified in controlled PMS treatment studies, ranging as high as 70 percent.[35,36] There is wide agreement that hormonal or psychotropic medications be prescribed only after two to three cycles of prospective symptom reports are obtained. However, there is little information about the effects of placebo treatment on these prospective symptom reports. We have found a significant decrease in overall symptom severity reported during the cycle following the first visit compared to the previsit cycle.[8] Because all patients are prescribed placebo capsules or vitamin B_6 (with no differences observed in patient global reports of improvement), placebo medication may be an important factor in this decrease.

Other researchers found that, even after three cycles of consistent prospective daily symptom reports, there was a significant decrease in symptoms during the first placebo-treated cycle.[6] It may be that placebo-treated cycles are essential for establishing a pretreatment symptom baseline.

PYRIDOXINE (VITAMIN B₆)

The theoretical rationale for vitamin B_6 administration was described by Abraham[37] and is based on earlier reports. In 1943 Biskind attributed premenstrual problems to estrogen excess from decreased liver clearance and reported successful treatment with the vitamin B complex.[38] Winston proposed that high estrogen levels during the luteal phase resulted in pyridoxine deficiency, decreased serotonin synthesis, and depressed mood.[39] Another rationale for use of pyridoxine is its possible role in increasing dopamine content in the hypothalamus and in increasing dopaminergic activity. Pyridoxine deficiencies were found in women taking oral contraceptives,[40] and depression was reduced with correction of the deficiency.

Studies of vitamin B_6 supplementation for premenstrual symptoms have given inconsistent results. One small, double-blind, placebo-controlled study in which 50 mg was given daily reported negative results.[41] Another placebo-controlled study used 50 mg daily and reported that luteal phase symptom scores were significantly lower in treated cycles than placebo cycles.[42] The sample was small and appeared to consist of women whose predominant symptoms were anxiety, tension, and edema; few indicated distress in the depression symptom cluster. Those who improved appeared to have moderate premenstrual symptoms, whereas women with severe symptoms were less likely to respond to vitamin B_6 treatment.

Williams et al. reported a sample of 434 PMS patients with 82 percent improved in the vitamin B_6 group and 70 percent improved in the placebo group as rated by physicians, a significant difference. However, patient reports of specific symptoms showed no significant differences between the vitamin B_6 or placebo groups.[43]

Possible side effects of vitamin B_6 at high dosage levels are nausea and dizziness. These side effects can usually be avoided by taking the medicine with other food or by lowering the dosage. There is evidence of peripheral neuropathy from pyridoxine abuse. Identified patients took daily doses of 4 to 6 g of pyridoxine—levels that were self-imposed on the theory that "more might be better."[44] The safety of 500 mg daily has subsequently been questioned. These reports demonstrate that megadoses of vitamins are not without risk and that long-term use should be carefully monitored.

MEDICATION

Because there is no single medication for the premenstrual syndrome, at present the only reliable approach to treatment depends on the isolation of specific symptoms. Therefore we believe that medication should not be used until isolation of symptoms, a psychological profile, and calendars are completed. At that point often the patient and clinician have more specific understanding of the problem.

We can divide the medications used to treat PMS into a number of categories. First are drugs that interfere with ovulation and produce cyclic changes. These drugs include oral contraceptive pills,[45,46] medroxyprogesterone acetate (Depo-Provera) or other long-acting progestins,[47,48] danazol,[49,50] or GnRH[51] analogues. All of these drugs at appropriate doses suppress ovulation. Cyclic estrogen fluctuation with follicle formation may occur with progestins (35 mg) or triphasic oral contraceptives, low doses of danazol, or GnRH analogues. Higher doses of danazol or GnRH analogues usually suppress even this estrogen fluctuation. These drugs are most successful for somatic cyclic symptoms particularly cramps, abdominal pain, or bloating. Each of these drugs does not help some patients or causes unpleasant side effects. It is important that the patient realize at the beginning of the therapy that the clinician may not find the "right" medication at first.

A specific symptom such as breast tenderness is often helped by low-dose danazol or bromocriptine (Parlodel). However, reassurance that these symptoms are not cancer but are normal fluctuations or a recommendation for changes in the diet may be all that is necessary. The decision rests on knowing the patient before prescribing medication.

Another group of medications are the diuretics. Traditionally, mild diuretics have been used to treat premenstrual feelings of water retention. First, it should be understood that premenstrual feelings of bloating are normal. Shifts in fluids may not be the only reason for this feeling, as gastrointestinal distention may also play a role. A few days of diuretics is often appreciated by the patient. However, there is mounting evidence that affective symptoms are not correlated with the changes in fluid. Therefore diuretics are in general unlikely to be helpful for the related affective symptoms of depression and anxiety.

Spironolactone is a mild diuretic with adrencortical and antiandrogen action. A number of investigators have found it helpful for affective symptoms. The role of this drug in PMS treatment is under investigation.[52]

The third group of drugs is more specifically used for affective symptoms, particularly irritability and mood swings. Potentially any of the tranquilizers could be used. Clinical experience with alprazolam, a benzodiazapine, has been good. Progesterone itself can be included in this category. Progesterone likely acts as a mild "tranquilizer," albeit a natural substance.[53] One study suggested that oral micronized progesterone therapy may be effective treatment for mood and some physical symptoms.[54] Vaginal progesterone suppositories have been inconsistently more effective than placebo and, when effective, likely to decrease irritability and hostility symptoms but not necessarily premenstrually.[55] Side effects of tranquilizer substances are well known and include depression.

Clinicians should be aware of the potential for abuse for all of these medications. For example, the patient seeking treatment for bloating may have such a distortion of body image that she will overutilize a diuretic in the effort to "feel" thin. Of course the abuse of tranquilizing drugs is well documented. Patients may increase the dosage of their medication to unsafe amounts when faced with severe situational problems.

SUMMARY

Of primary importance in the treatment of PMS is appropriate diagnostic assessment. Critical evaluation of (1) the existence of premenstrual symptoms distinct from other psychological disorders and systemic disease; (2) the types of symptoms reported; and (3) the severity of symptoms premenstrually in comparison to the postmenstrual baseline are necessary for proper diagnosis and treatment.

Those patients who respond best to conservative therapy, including supportive counseling, nutrition and exercise modifications, and stress management education, are most often those patients with few follicular phase symptoms. These patients also have a high rate of placebo response. It is with this group that the clinician gynecologist can be most helpful.

Patients who are symptomatic postmenstrually, even if there is a significant increase in symptoms premenstrually, appear to be optimally treated for a primary psychological problem by a qualified mental health professional. These women are probably not helped in the long term by treatment with hormonal or psychotropic medication for premenstrual symptoms. Such patients require careful evaluation of symptom calendars and a psychological assessment during the follicular phase. With this information, a thoughtful, successful referral for psychological treatment can be made.

ACKNOWLEDGMENTS

We thank Natalie Sondheimer, MSS, for her editorial assistance and Joby M. Jackson for typing the manuscript.

REFERENCES

1. Crowley WF, Filicori M, Spratt D, et al: The physiology of gonadotropin releasing hormone (GnRH) secretion in men and women. Recent Prog Horm Res 41:473, 1985.
2. Woods NJ, Most A, Dery GK; Prevalence of perimenopausal symptoms. Am J Public Health 72:1257, 1982
3. Blume E: Premenstrual syndromes, depression links. JAMA 249:2864, 1983
4. Rubinow DR, Roy-Byrne P: Premenstrual syndromes: overview from a methodological perspective. Am J Psychiatry 141:163, 1984
5. Abplanalp JA, Donnelly AF, Rose RM: Psychoendocrinology of the menstrual cycle. I. Enjoyment of daily activities and moods. Psychosom Med 41:587, 1979
6. Metcalf MC, Hudson SM: The premenstrual syndrome: selection of women for treatment trials. J Psychosom Res 29:631, 1985
7. Hamilton JA, Parry BL, Alagna S, et al: Premenstrual mood changes: a guide to evaluation and treatment. Psychiatr Ann 14:426, 1984
8. Freeman EW, Rickels K, Sondheimer SJ, Scharlop B: Diagnostic classifications from daily symptom ratings of women who seek treatment for premenstrual symptoms. Submitted
9. Hargrove JT, Abraham GE: The incidence of premenstrual tension in a gynecologic clinic. Reprod Med 27:721, 1982

10. Freeman EW, Sondheimer SJ, Weinbaum PJ, Rickels K: Evaluating premenstrual symptoms in medical practice. Obstet Gynecol 65:500, 1985
11. Hamilton M: Development of a rating scale for primary depressive illness. Br J Soc Clinic Psychol 6:278, 1967
12. Hamilton M: The assessment of anxiety states by rating. Br J Med Psychol 32:50, 1959
13. Endicott J, Spitzer RL: A diagnostic interview: the schedule for affective disorders and schizophrenia. Arch Gen Psychiatry 35:837, 1978
14. Diagnostic and Statistical Manual of Mental Disorders. 3rd Ed. American Psychiatric Association, Washington, DC, 1980
15. Dahlstrom WG, Welsh GS: An MMPI Handbook. University of Minnesota Press, Minneapolis, 1960
16. Sondheimer SJ, Freeman EW, Scharlop B, Rickels K: Hormonal changes in premenstrual syndrome. Psychosomatics 26:803, 1985
17. Dennerstein L, Spencer-Gardner C, Brown JB, et al: Premenstrual tension-hormonal profiles. J Psychol Obstet Gynecol 3:37, 1984
18. Andersch B, Abrahamsson L, Wendestam C, et al: Hormone profile in PMT: effects of bromocriptine and diuretics. Clin Endocrinol (Oxf) 11:657, 1979
19. Backstrom T, Sanders D, Leask R, et al. Mood, sexuality, hormones and the menstrual cycle. II. Hormone levels and their relationship to the premenstrual syndrome. Psychosom Med 45:503, 1983
20. Evans JA, Austin C, Speroff L: The effect of non-exercise related stress on the menstrual cycle: a preliminary report. Abstract 221. In: Abstracts of the 1986 Meeting, American Fertility Society
21. Clare AW: Hormones, behavior and the menstrual cycle. J Psychosom Res 29:225, 1985
22. Klaiber EL, Kobayashi U, Broverman DM, et al: Plasma monoamine oxidase activity in regularly menstruating women and in amenorrheic women receiving cyclic treatment with estrogens and a progestin. J Clin Endocrinol Metab 33:630, 1971
23. Klaiber EL, Broverman D, Vogel W, et al: Estrogens and CNS function: EEG, cognition, and depression. In Friedman R (ed): Behavior and the Menstrual Cycle. Marcel Dekker, New York, 1982
24. Vogel W, Broverman DM, Klaiber EL: EEG responses in regularly menstruating women and in amenorrheic women treated with ovarian hormones. Science 172: 388, 1971
25. Jewelewicz R: The role of endogenous opioid peptides in control of the menstrual cycle. Fertil Steril 42:683, 1984
26. Shoupe D, Montz FJ, Lobo RA: The effects of estrogen and progestin on endogenous opioid activity in oophorectomized women. J Clin Endocrinol Metab 60:178, 1985
27. Rausch J, Janowsky D, Risch SC, et al: Hormonal and neurotransmitter hypotheses of premenstrual tension. Psychopharmacol Bull 18:26, 1982
28. Adams PW, Rose DP, Folkard J, et al: Effects of pyridoxine hydrochloride (vitamin B-6) upon depression associated with oral contraceptives. Lancet 1:897, 1973
29. Lahmeyer HW, Miller M, DeLeon-Jones F: Anxiety and mood fluctuation during the normal menstrual cycle. Psychosom Med 44:183, 1982
30. Faratian B, Gaspar A, O'Brien PM, et al: Premenstrual syndrome: weight, abdominal swelling, and perceived body image. Am J Obstet Gynecol 150:200, 1984
31. Reid RL, Greenaway-Coates A, Hahn PM: Oral glucose tolerance during the men-

strual cycle in normal women and women with alleged premenstrual hypogly-cemic attacks: effects of naloxone. J Clin Endocrinol Metab 62:1167, 1986

32. Wald A, Van Thiel D, Hoechstetter L, et al: Gastrointestinal transit: the effect of the menstrual cycle. Gastroenterology 80:1497, 1983

33. Levitt DB, Freeman EW, Sondheimer SJ, Rickels K: Group support in the treatment of PMS. J Psychosoc Nurs 26:23, 1986

34. Freeman EW, Sondheimer SJ, Rickels K, Weinbaum PJ: PMS treatment approaches and progesterone therapy. Psychosomatics 26:811, 1985

35. Green J: recent trends in the treatment of premenstrual syndrome: a critical review. In Friedman RC (ed). Behavior and the Menstrual Cycle. Marcel Dekker, New York, 1983

36. Harrison WM, Endicott J, Rabkin JG, et al: Treatment of premenstrual dysphoric changes: clinical outcome and methodological implications. Psychopharmacol Bull 20:118, 1984

37. Abraham GE: Nutritional factors in the etiology of the premenstrual tension syndromes. J Reprod Med 28:446, 1983

38. Biskind M: Nutritional deficiency in the etiology of menorrhagia, metrorrhia, cystic mastitis and premenstrual tension: treatment with vitamin B complex. J Clin Endocrinol Metab 3:227, 1943

39. Winston F: Oral contraceptives, pyridoxine and depression. Am J Psychiatry 130:1217, 1973

40. Price JM, Thornton MJ, Mueller LM: Tryptophan metabolism in women using steroid hormones for ovulation control. Am J Clin Nutr 20:452, 1967

41. Stokes J, Mendels J: Pyridoxine and premenstrual tension. Lancet 1:1177, 1972

42. Abraham GE, Hargrove JT: Effect of vitamin B-6 on premenstrual symptomatology in women with premenstrual tension syndromes: a double-blind crossover study. Infertility 3:155, 1980

43. Williams MJ, Harris RI, Dean BC: Controlled trial of pyridoxine in the premenstrual syndrome. J Int Med Res 13:174, 1985

44. Schaumberg H, Kaplan J, Windebank A, et al: Sensory neuropathy from pyridoxine abuse. N Engl J Med 309:445, 1983

45. Cullberg J: Mood changes and menstrual symptoms with different gestagen/estrogen combinations. Acta Psychiatr Scand [Suppl] 236:1, 1972

46. Coppen AJ, Milna HB, Outram DH, et al: Dytide, norethisterone and a placebo in the premenstrual syndrome—a double-blind comparison. Clin Trials J 6:33, 1969

47. Taylor RW: The treatment of premenstrual tension with dydrogesterone. Curr Med Res Opin 4: suppl. 4, 16, 1977

48. Jordheim O: The premenstrual syndrome. Acta Obstet Gynecol Scand 51:77, 1972

49. Gilmore DH, Hawthorne RJS, Hart DM: Danazol for premenstrual syndrome: a preliminary report of a placebo-controlled double-blind study. J Int Med Res 13: 129, 1985

50. Watts JF, Edwards RL, Butt WR: Treatment of premenstrual syndrome using danazol: preliminary report of a placebo-controlled, double-blind, dose ranging study. J Int Med Res 13:127, 1985

51. Muse KN, Cetel NS, Futterman LA, Yen SSC: The premenstrual syndrome: effects of medical ovariectomy. N Engl J Med 311:1345, 1984

52. O'Brien PMS, Craven D, Selby C, et al: Treatment of premenstrual syndrome by spironolactone. Br J Obstet Gynaecol 86:142, 1979

53. Majewska MD, Harrison NL, Schwartz RD, et al: Steroid hormone metabolites are barbiturate-like modulators of the GABA receptor. Science 232:1004, 1986

54. Dennerstein L, Spencer-Gardner L, Gotts G, et al: Progesterone and the premenstrual syndrome: a double-blind crossover trial. Br Med J 290:1017, 1985
55. Maddocks S, Kahn P, Moller F, Reid R: A double-blind placebo controlled trial of progesterone vaginal suppositories in the treatment of premenstrual syndrome. Am J Obstet Gynecol 54:573, 1986

7

Current Views and the Beta-Endorphin Hypothesis

C. James Chuong
Carolyn B. Coulam

Since 1931, when Frank[1] first described cyclic changes occurring before menses, the premenstrual syndrome (PMS) has been accepted as a complex of symptoms characterized by psychological changes including irritability, aggression, tension, anxiety, and depression, and by somatic changes attributed to fluid retention such as the feeling of being bloated, weight increase, edema, breast tenderness, and headaches before menses. Because these symptoms have been implicated in marital discord,[2] child abuse,[3] criminal behavior,[4] absenteeism, and work inefficiency[5] attention has been drawn to understanding the pathophysiologic features of PMS in the hope of finding an effective treatment. The social and economic concerns are enhanced by estimates of the prevalence of premenstrual symptoms in 70 to 90 percent of the female population and incapacitation in 20 to 40 percent.[6] Because of the increased role of women in the work force, the impact of PMS is of economic significance, and it has received increased attention by both the lay and the medical communities. However, to date, the lack of universally accepted criteria for the diagnosis, the obscurity of its etiology, and contradictory results of medication trials indicate that PMS continues to be an unsolved problem. This chapter addresses the current conceptualization of PMS and presents current research data.

ENDOCRINE ASPECTS OF PMS

Studies establishing the relation between cyclic symptoms and endocrine changes and identifying hormones whose levels vary during the luteal phase have been reported. Serum hormone concentrations have been determined during the follicular and luteal phases in both controls and PMS patients. There have been no consistent significant differences between the groups in terms of the levels of prolactin, growth hormone, estrogen, progesterone, sex hormone binding globulin (SHBG), thyroxine, thyroid-stimulating hormone, testosterone, dehydroepiandrosterone sulfate (DHEA-S), and aldosterone.[7-9] Circadian secretory profiles of prolactin and growth hormone have also failed to distinguish PMS patients.[10] In terms of ovarian sex steroids, although some studies have found serum estrogen levels and the estrogen:progesterone ratio in PMS patients higher than those in controls during the luteal phase,[9,11] other studies showed either no difference or lower estrogen levels after ovulation.[12,13] Data on progesterone deficiency during the luteal phase are equally inconclusive.[9,13] Furthermore, SHBG was noted to be either unchanged[14] or significantly lower[15] in the symptomatic group. Elevated levels of gonadotropins—follicle-stimulating hormone (FSH) and luteinizing hormone (LH)—have been reported but are presumably related to elevated estrogen levels.[13,14] Finally, although Charvat and Holececk have shown premenstrual elevations of antidiuretic hormone (ADH) in some patients,[16] these results must be confirmed before any conclusions can be drawn.

The search for a hormonal cause of PMS led to cortisol, as it is known to relate to psychological symptoms. About 50 percent of depressed patients are resistant to the cortisol-suppressing effect of dexamethasone. This dexamethasone suppression test (DST) has attracted considerable attention as a possible biologic marker for depression.[17] Although depression is one of the main symptoms of PMS, to date there have been conflicting findings regarding cortisol levels in these women. Steiner et al.[10] did not find significant differences in the circadian secretory profiles of cortisol between controls and patients, whereas Muse et al.[18] demonstrated higher cortisol levels (lack of suppression or positive DST) in patients compared with controls with no early escape. However, Sondheimer et al.[8] have pointed out that the lack of specificity limits the usefulness of the DST in PMS.

In view of the above data, it seems likely that patterns of hormonal changes throughout the menstrual cycle rather than point hormone levels can identify patients with PMS. Unfortunately, it is difficult to measure these changes. Based on the above findings, it is clear that the routine use of peripheral hormonal tests for patients with premenstrual complaints is not only costly but also not indicated at this time. However, a new area which needs further study is the β-endorphin (β-EP), as we have found that lower levels of β-EP during the luteal phase may be associated with premenstrual symptoms (see Pathophysiology, below).

PSYCHOLOGICAL ASPECTS OF PMS

In 1985 PMS was classified as "premenstrual dysphoric disorder" and was proposed for inclusion in the revised *Diagnostic and Statistical Manual III (DSM-III-R)* as a mental disorder. After further discussion, in 1986 the Board of Trustees of the American Psychiatric Association (APA) accepted the recommendation of the APA work group to change the name of "premenstrual dysphoric disorder" to "periluteal phase dysphoric disorder," then to "late luteal phase dysphoric disorder"; they finally placed this diagnosis in the appendix rather than the text of the manual.

Those who proposed PMS as a psychiatric disorder emphasized that the principal symptoms of PMS are "psychological and behavioral rather than physical, and the differential diagnosis is with the other mental disorders rather than with physical disorders." However, PMS is a multifactorial psychoneuroendocrine disorder.[6] The degree of severity and presentation of various symptoms is modified and/or aggravated by other factors, e.g., diet, exercise, and stress-related factors from the environment such as those related to job, family, and school. The idea that PMS is psychological and behavioral rather than physical is difficult to accept despite the fact that psychological symptoms such as mood swings, tension, anxiety, irritability, depression, etc. are part of the manifestations. We also disagree with the PMS diagnosis criteria proposed by the psychiatric group with the emphasis on mood and behavior as opposed to somatic symptoms such as abdominal bloating, weight gain, finger swelling, headache, hot flashes, bowel habit changes, etc.

Another confounding factor is that the PMS population is not homogeneous. Heterogeneity is found in the kind of symptoms, the timing of symptoms, and the psychological status. Typical patients complain equally of mood, behavior, and somatic symptoms, but symptoms in one category may predominate for some patients. Symptoms typically disappear within 2 days after the onset of the menstrual flow, but Reid[19] has reported four different temporal patterns of PMS, one with symptoms lasting throughout menstruation. An attempt has been made to distinguish two subgroups on the basis of psychological status using the Minnesota Multiphasic Personality Inventory (MMPI).[20] The MMPI was given to 20 women with PMS and 20 women without PMS during the follicular and luteal phases of the menstrual ccyle[20] (Table 7-1). Women without PMS had no clinically significant MMPI changes during their cycles. Women with PMS, however, had many statistically and clinically significant changes in MMPI response patterns over their cycles. Less effective psychological functioning and increased psychological stress were observed during the luteal phase compared with the follicular phase. Median scores on all scales [except 5(Mf) and 9(Ma)] were significantly increased during the luteal phase (Fig. 7-1).[20] PMS patients were also found to have more feelings of worry, tension, anxiety, and interpersonal oversensitivity than the control group. Keye et al.[21] has reported similar results. These data suggest the existence of two PMS subgroups. The first has cyclic variations from completely normal MMPI values during the follicular phase to significantly dysfunctional levels during the luteal phase. The second has psychological stress and dysfunction throughout the cycle that are significantly greater than those in women without PMS and that are exacerbated during the luteal phase. From 25 to 50 percent of our PMS patients had MMPI profiles that indicated a need for further evaluation of mental health, e.g., a psychiatric consultation. These patients may have had a chronic depressive disorder or other affective disorder, as well as premenstrual exacerbation of symptoms, or have had typical PMS initially but developed a chronic dys-

TABLE 7-1. MINNESOTA MULTIPHASIC PERSONALITY INVENTORY MEDIAN T SCORES[a] BY DAY OF CYCLE AND MEDIAN INTRACYCLE CHANGE IN T SCORES FOR PATIENTS WITH PMS AND CONTROL SUBJECTS

| Scale | Day 7 (Follicular) | | | Day 25 (Luteal) | | | Day 7 to Day 25 (Intracycle Changes) | |
	Control (median)	PMS (median)	Control vs. PMS (rank-sum p value)	Control (median)	PMS (median)	Control vs. PMS (rank-sum p value)	Control (median)	PMS (median)
L	51	46	>0.20	46	46[b]	>0.2000	0	2
F	46[c]	51	0.043	39[c]	57[c]	<0.0001	0	-7[c]
K	57[c]	52	0.12	59[c]	44[b]	<0.0001	-1	9[c]
1(Hs)	45[c]	50	0.056	46[b]	51	0.0039	0	-2[b]
2(D)	44[c]	51	0.013	41[c]	60[c]	<0.0001	0	-9[c]
3(Hy)	53	51	>0.20	50	60[c]	0.0023	0	-7[c]
4(Pd)	54	53	>0.20	51	61[c]	0.0009	0	-6[c]
5(Mf)	52	45	>0.20	47	44	>0.2000	2	2
6(Pa)	48[d]	56[b]	0.0017	46[d]	61[c]	0.0001	0	-6[d]
7(Pt)	46[d]	53	0.016	47[b]	60[c]	0.0008	-2	-6[c]
8(Sc)	46	51	>0.20	48	52[b]	0.0250	-2	-7[c]
9(Ma)	50	54	>0.20	48	55	0.0590	0	-2
0(Si)	40[c]	45	0.10	38[c]	54	0.0002	2	-5[c]

[a] All T scores are based on the contemporary adult norms (which have a median of 50).
[b] Signed-rank test of T score different from 50 (zero for day 7 to day 25) is significant with $0.02 < p < 0.05$.
[c] Signed-rank test of T score different from 50 (zero for day 7 to day 25) is significant with $p < 0.01$.
[d] Signed-rank test of T score different from 50 (zero for day 7 to day 25) is significant with $0.01 < p < 0.02$.

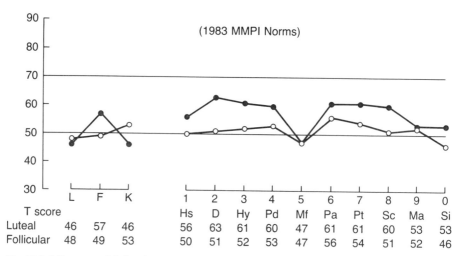

Fig. 7-1 Minnesota Multiphasic Personality Inventory (MMPI) profile on day 7 (follicular phase) and day 25 (luteal phase) of the menstrual cycle for 20 women with premenstrual syndrome.

phoric disorder or other psychopathology throughout the menstrual cycle after suffering with cyclic symptoms for a significant length of time. In this regard Friedman et al.[22] has postulated an etiologic role of sensitization to monthly mood changes over years of cycles. Although the second group of patients may be classified as having psychiatric as well as physical illness, they should not be considered as having purely psychiatric illness, and the evaluation needs to be conducted appropriately.[23] Different treatment approaches are likely to be needed for different subgroups of PMS patients.

PATHOPHYSIOLOGY

The pathophysiology of PMS remains elusive. The frequent discrepancy between subjective and objective findings contributes to the problem, as does the heterogeneity of reactions and range of severity that women report. Numerous hypotheses regarding pathophysiology have been proposed since Frank first described premenstrual tension in 1931. These hypotheses have been reviewed by Reid and Yen,[6] who examined the relative validity of existing hypotheses and concluded that PMS was a multifactorial psychoneuroendocrine disorder. Current hypotheses are presented and discussed along with recent data. The hypothesis that cyclic variations in neuropeptides activity during the menstrual cycle are related to various premenstrual changes is presented.

FLUID RETENTION

It has long been suggested that PMS might be related to hormones responsible for fluid retention, and as a result diuretics remain one of the most commonly prescribed treatments for PMS. Although it is widely believed that premenstrual weight gain is a normal occurrence caused by salt and water retention,[24] no consistent weight increase is noted in asymptomatic women.[25] Furthermore, patients with PMS do not show consistent weight changes either, nor is there a correlation between weight and symptoms.[26] Although weight gain does not seem to occur, redistribution of fluid does, and several hormones have been suggested as specific etiologic agents. The ovarian steroids affect the renin–angiotensin–aldosterone axis. Estrogen causes sodium and water retention, whereas progesterone has opposite effects, which may result in a compensatory release of aldosterone during the luteal phase. Although aldosterone is elevated during the luteal phase of the menstrual cycle, no significant differences in aldosterone levels have been noted between PMS patients and controls.[9]

Another factor that might contribute to the fluid retention is atrial natriuretic factor (ANF). Its infusion produces an increase in urinary output and natriuresis. Atrial distention appears to be a stimulus for ANF release. In a preliminary report on PMS, Davidson et al.[27] showed no changes in ANF or plasma renin activity between the follicular and luteal phases. Angiotensin II levels are elevated during the second half of the menstrual cycle in normal women, but there have been no studies of angiotensin II levels in women with PMS. A few studies have suggested that ADH may contribute to premenstrual fluid retention. Charvat and Holececk showed that some of their patients had elevated ADH levels premenstrually,[16] but ADH levels have not been measured in patients with severe premenstrual edema. Cortisol has some mineralocorticoid effects, and its increase may contribute fluid retention; however, no significant changes have been noted in cortisol levels between the follicular and luteal phases.[10]

Some PMS patients perceive that fluid retention is related to the severity of symptoms, even with the absence of weight change. However, studies assessing total exchangeable sodium and total body water have failed to uncover a pattern of fluid retention in most PMS patients.[28] Although the above findings do not support a fluid retention hypothesis, a mechanism by which there is redistribution of fluid into specific compartments remains feasible.

HYPERPROLACTINEMIA

Because of its direct effect on the breasts, its relation to stress through dopamine metabolism, and its possible role in causing fluid retention, prolactin has been considered to be associated with PMS. However, several studies have shown that patients with PMS do not have higher prolactin levels[8,10] than controls, and patients with hyperprolactinemia do not have premenstrual changes.

PROSTAGLANDINS

Prostaglandins (PGs) have been implicated in the etiology of PMS and are produced in varying amounts in response to changing levels of estrogens and progesterones. They exert sedative effects on the central nervous system and affect both aldosterone activity and ADH release, but neither E-series nor F-series prostaglandins[29] vary significantly during the menstrual cycle. Preliminary reports on PMS show significantly lower levels of PGE_2 and $PGF_{2\alpha}$ throughout the menstrual cycle, which may indicate an excess formation of PGE_1.[30]

Both prostaglandin precursors and prostaglandin inhibitors have been used to treat PMS. The oil of evening primrose contains dihomo-γ-linoleic acid and linoleic acid, dietary precursors of PGE_1 and PGE_2, respectively, and has been used to treat PMS. Prostaglandin synthetase inhibitors (the nonsteroid anti-inflammatory drugs) cure dysmenorrhea, or menstrual cramps, that may overlap with premenstrual symptoms, and these drugs have also been used to treat PMS. This fact suggests that if premenstrual changes are mediated to some extent by prostaglandins it may be the balance between the various prostaglandins, rather than an overall increase or decrease, that is involved.

HYPOGLYCEMIA

Food craving is a common complaint of women with PMS. This problem combined with other symptoms such as fatigue, dizziness, and cold sweats, has led some workers to consider the possibility of reactive hypoglycemia as a contributing factor. Early studies showed evidence of a flattened glucose tolerance curve and reduced insulin receptor concentration during the luteal phase.[31] However, plasma glucose levels less than 50 mg/dl are rarely observed during the time "hypoglycemia attacks" are reported by PMS patients. Nevertheless, Reid et al.[32] reported the existence of luteal phase abnormalities in glucose metabolism, including elevated fasting plasma glucose and glucagon and increased glucose and insulin responses to an oral glucose load in women with premenstrual "hypoglycemic attacks" compared to normal women. They also observed greater rates of decreased glucose levels in patients compared to controls and concluded that altered glucose metabolism leading to exaggerated glucose swings during the luteal phase might account for premenstrual hypoglycemic symptoms.[32] Naltrexone failed to alter those abnormalities,[33] and whether endogenous opiate peptides are involved in the regulation of pancreatic islet cell activity needs further study. The fact that premenstrual symptoms are not confined to times when hypoglycemia is likely suggests that there is not a causal relation, although a concurrence of these conditions cannot be ruled out.

PROGESTERONE DEFICIENCY AND WITHDRAWAL

Frank was the first to propose that PMS was due to excess estrogen.[1] Israel and others[34,35] asserted that an unopposed estrogenic effect, due to deficient progesterone production, was linked to PMS, based on luteal phase steroid levels, endometrial biopsies, and vaginal smears in PMS patients. On the other hand, several reports of adequate corpus luteal function in affected women suggested that progesterone withdrawal, rather than progesterone deficiency, caused PMS, as symptoms are known to be maximal as progesterone levels decrease during the late luteal phase. The rate of fall of progesterone levels has been implicated as an etiologic factor.

VITAMIN B₆ DEFICIENCY

During the 1940s Biskind and Biskind[36] postulated a deficiency of vitamin B complex as the cause of excess estrogen in PMS patients. Administration of vitamin B_6 was reported to result in clinical improvement in PMS symptoms. However, it was noted that women with severe vitamin B_6 deficiency had normal estrogen metabolism,[37] and subsequently the therapy lost popularity. It has again been suggested that vitamin B_6 therapy may be beneficial owing to its regulation of the production of brain biogenic amines. Mood and behavior are influenced by excitatory and inhibitory biogenic amines present in the central nervous system (CNS). Asberg reported that 40 percent of a group of depressed patients with lower levels of 5-hydroxyindoleacetic acid, the breakdown product of serotonin, had attempted suicide.[38] Several PMS symptoms represent an excitatory state of the CNS, and the aim of treatment is to lower excitatory biogenic amines and to increase inhibitory ones.

Vitamin B_6 is thought to be unique in its ability to perform this function. Not only does it increase inhibitory amines such as dopamine and serotonin, it also increases the conversion of CNS-active excitatory amino acids to the corresponding inhibitory amino acids by functioning as a coenzyme. Therefore the overall effect of vitamin B_6 is an increased ratio of inhibitory/excitatory amines. Such an effect would result in sedation.[39]

β-ENDORPHIN WITHDRAWAL

A number of substances have been shown to influence behavior, including neurotransmitters and small peptides with opiate receptor activity. Such peptides, termed *endorphins*, are derived from enzymatic cleavage of a larger peptide (91 amino acids), β-lipotropin. High concentrations of endorphins and opiate receptor binding sites have been found on dopaminergic neurons within the basal medial hypothalamus, suggesting that endorphins may play a mediatory or modulatory role in these neuronal functions.[40]

Endorphin and estrogen levels have been shown to covary. Progesterone is also associated with an increase in endogenous opiate peptide activity.[41,42] During the luteal phase of the menstrual cycle, when symptoms of PMS occur, plasma levels of estrogen add progesterone rise as the corpus luteum functions and then fall as the corpus luteum regresses. During the latter part of pregnancy, when estrogen and progesterone levels are high, elevated endorphin levels are also observed. Postpartum, when estrogen and progesterone levels fall, endorphin levels also fall.[43] In manic-depressive patients the cerebrospinal fluid endorphin levels have been noted to be elevated during the manic stage. In patients with puerperal psychosis, endorphin levels have been found to be elevated during the acute drug-free stage. During a later symptom-free stage, after treatment with electroconvulsive treatment and/or neuroleptics, the endorphin levels were within the normal range.[44] These observations suggested that some of the psychological symptoms of PMS might be related to steroid hormone or opiate withdrawal.

Experiments with naloxone, an opiate receptor antagonist, provide more evidence in support of the endogenous opiate hypothesis. Naloxone was found to produce symptoms similar to those of PMS when it was administered in high doses to normal volunteers.[45] More evidence comes from observations of menopausal-like hot flashes in PMS patients by Reid et al.[46] They noted the subjective awareness of chills and sweats at the time of other PMS symptoms in 72 percent of 120 women with PMS. The onset of premenstrual chills and sweating was close to the onset of other premenstrual symptoms in most individuals. Objective measurements in one subject revealed episodes of chills and sweating to be linked to falling skin resistance, rising finger temperature, and LH pulses. Opiate withdrawal may be accompanied by decreasing estrogen action and may be linked to hot flash activity in some PMS patients.[46] Acute withdrawal of opiate inhibition of biogenic amine systems, may lead to rebound hyperactivity of neuronal pathways owing to slowly acquired receptor supersensitivity, resulting in irritability, anxiety, tension, and aggression. Variations in the degree and duration of opiate exposure and the rapidity of withdrawal might account for differences in the severity of premenstrual symptoms from one cycle to another.[6,47]

The endogenous β-EP levels have been shown to peak at midcycle with no obvious difference between the follicular phase and the luteal phase in normal ovulatory women. In human subjects intravenous β-EP caused a decrease in the LH level, and the opiate receptor antagonist naloxone caused an increase in LH concentration.[48] Therefore it is suggested that there is a chronic inhibitory effect of β-EP on gonadotropin secretion. Some PMS patients were noted to have a blunted LH response to naloxone during both follicular and luteal phases. A higher plasma FSH level was also noted during the early and midluteal phase in some PMS patients.[49] Both studies indicated that a deficiency of central opioid activity may be associated with PMS symptoms. We found that PMS patients have lower levels of plasma endorphin during the luteal phase of the menstrual cycle compared to their own levels during the follicular phase and compared to controls during the luteal phase (Fig. 7-2). None of the other neuropeptides investigated—including neurotensin, human pancreatic peptide, vasoactive intestinal polypeptide, gastrin, and bombesin-like immunoreactivity—showed significant changes.[50]

Because the blood–brain barrier is relatively impermeable to the passage of anterior pituitary hormones, including β-EP,[51] it has been argued that there is no relation between peripheral and central levels of β-EP. Currently available techniques do not afford access to the central site of synthesis and secretion of β-EP, thereby allowing direct measurement of this neuropeptide in patients with PMS. However, studies have demonstrated a parallel increase in pituitary content and circulating levels of β-EP in genetically obese rats.[52] Having observed the changes in peripheral β-EP levels in PMS, we propose that parallel changes in peripheral and central β-EP may occur and that the premenstrual decrease of β-EP peripherally may reflect a decrease in central levels of β-EP and may be responsible for the PMS symptom complex.

Several factors may alter peripheral β-EP levels, e.g., psychiatric disorders, levels of activity, food intake, diurnal changes. Our previous findings were based on a single blood sample obtained with the patient in a fasting stage between 7:30 a.m. and 9:30 a.m. on days 7 and 25 of the menstrual cycle. However, levels of activity may vary throughout the day. Whereas some patients restrict their activity because of an inability to go to work or school, a tendency to stay away from others, and somatic changes such as sore breasts or rheumatic complaints, others increase their activity because of irritability, aggression, anger and arguing with others, etc. Whether PMS patients have persistently lower levels of plasma endorphin throughout the day premenstrually is currently under investigation.

EVALUATION OF PREMENSTRUAL COMPLAINTS

Certain practical considerations need to be kept in mind during the evaluation of premenstrual changes. The protocol of our PMS clinic appears in Figure 7-3.

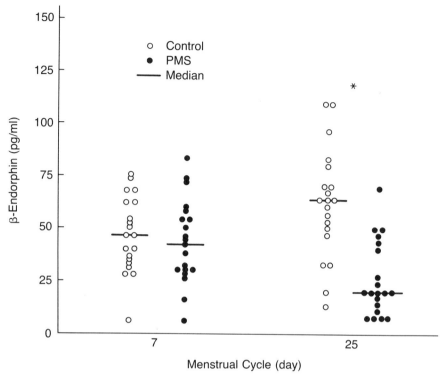

Fig. 7-2 The β-EP levels for control subjects and PMS patients on days 7 and 25 of the menstrual cycle.* The PMS group is significantly different from the control group (p = 0.0001) on day 25. (Chuong CJ, Coulam CB, Kao PC, et al. Neuropeptide levels in premenstrual syndrome. Fertil Steril 44:760, 1985. Reproduced with permission of the publisher, The American Fertility Society).

1. It is important to determine if the patient's complaints are actually postovulatory and premenstrual. The character of the symptoms is probably less important than the timing. It is critical for the diagnosis of PMS that symptoms occur specifically during the luteal phase of the cycle and that there is a symptom-free period of at least a week following cessation of menstruation. Symptoms continuing after the second day of the menstrual cycle are not generally considered PMS.

2. There are still no uniformly accepted criteria for the diagnosis of PMS, and we have to depend on the patient's subjective report. Prospective recording of symptoms using a daily diary, specific mood assessment charts, or specific visual analogue scales is much more predictive of premenstrual changes than are retrospective reports, which tend to overdiagnose PMS.

3. The diagnosis is frequently inaccurate. Premenstrual changes are confused with other gynecologic and/or psychiatric problems. The evaluation should include not only a detailed history but the formulation of a differential diagnosis of each complaint and a thorough physical and psychological exam-

PMS Clinic Protocol

I. Initial visit
  A. History and physical examination
  B. Psychiatric consultation if necessary
  C. Questionnaire
    1. Menstrual distress questionnaire (MDQ)
    2. PMS questionnaire
    3. Minnesota Multiphasic Personality Inventory (MMPI) — optional
    4. PMS daily diary
    5. Basal body temperature (BBT)
  D. Laboratory tests
    1. Prolactin
    2. Total thyroxine
    3. Fasting blood sugar
    4. β-endorphin, vitamins, minerals, etc. for the purpose of study
II. Second visit (in 1–2 months)
  A. Review questionnaires and BBT
  B. Laboratory tests results
  C. Diagnosis

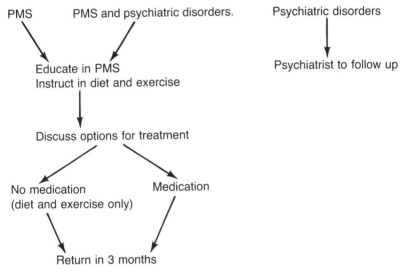

Fig. 7-3 PMS clinic protocol.

ination, with laboratory and radiologic examinations and referrals when appropriate.[21] It is particularly important to differentiate PMS from psychiatric diagnoses, e.g., affective disorders, which may be exacerbated during the premenstrual phase.

The Menstrual Distress Questionnaire (MDQ) has been validated in three populations without PMS, and normative values for the postmenstrual week and the premenstrual week have been described.[53] Women whose scores on the MDQ were ≤80 on day 7 or ≥95 on day 25 of the menstrual cycle were considered to have PMS. Those whose scores were ≤ 80 on day 7 and < 95 on day 25 were considered not to have PMS. Those whose scores were > 80 on day 7 were referred for psychiatric consultation. The reliability of this questionnaire was tested by having it completed for three consecutive cycles.[20] The PMS questionnaire contains 30 questions with a 1 to 4 scale, which was modified from Steiner et al.[54] Its validation is currently being conducted.

Although there is no relation between the serum prolactin, thyroxine, or glucose levels and PMS, hyperprolactinemia, thyroid dysfunction, and diabetes mellitus can cause somatic and affective symptoms that are occasionally mistaken for PMS unless appropriate testing is obtained.

MANAGEMENT

Most women can cope with mild premenstrual changes, but for those with moderate or severe symptoms the physical discomfort and emotional instability can be stressful. Traditionally, PMS was viewed as "just part of being a woman." Only recently has the medical community and lay public become sensitive to this issue. Treatment presents a challenge because of the many variables involved. Our approach is shown in Figure 7-3.

GENERAL APPROACH

Education

Discussion with patients and their families about the nature of the syndrome is important. Knowing that symptoms are cyclic and hormone-related rather than "all in the head" can provide relief. Patients should be informed that PMS is a physiologic phenomenon that occurs in many healthy, productive women. Sources of stress from the environment, weather, job, family, school, etc. that aggravate premenstrual changes should be identified. Of note are seasonal premenstrual and affective changes, which have recently been described. Strategies for coping with these factors may then become apparent. The patients need to learn to expect when the symptoms will occur and so avoid making important decisions, or performing stressful duties during that time. Family members also need to anticipate the premenstruum and help patients to live through the "bad days."

Diet and Exercise

Eating regular small meals, decreasing the intake of salts, fats, sugar, and caffeine, and increasing exercise are helpful. Foods that are high in refined sugars and fats and that are highly processed are avoided. Food made from whole grains, legumes, seeds and nuts, vegetables, fruits, and vetetable oils are encouraged. The PMS Prevention Diet [54a] emphasizes whole fresh foods (Table 7-2).

A study from Finland revealed that women who participated in sports experience less premenstrual anxiety than nonathletic women.[55] How exercise

TABLE 7-2. THE PMS PREVENTION DIET

Foods made from whole grains

Whole grains (including wheat, corn, barley, oats, rye, millet, buckwheat, and brown rice) are complex carbohydrates, capable of stabilizing your blood sugar and helping tremendously to eliminate premenstrual sugar craving. They contain excellent sources of protein, fiber, vitamins B and E, and various minerals. They can be prepared in a variety of ways. Also try the following foods made from whole grain: cereals, bread, crackers (especially brown rice cakes), pancakes and waffles, and even pasta.

Legumes

Lentils, kidney beans, pinto beans, mung beans, garbanzo beans, adzuki beans, green peas, and the other members of the legume family can be used in many ways. They can become bases for thick soups. They can be eaten in salads or used in dips and casseroles. When eaten with grains they form a complete protein comparable to that in eggs or meat.

Seeds and nuts

Seeds and nuts are excellent sources of protein. They should be either dry-roasted or raw and unsalted. They are very high in calories so quantities consumed should be moderate if premenstrual weight gain is a problem for you. If you have acne, eat only very small amounts.

Vegetables

Most vegetables are rich in vitamins and minerals. Particularly good for women with PMS are root vegetables such as rutabagas, carrots, turnips, parsnips, and leafy green vegetables such as kale, collard, and mustard greens.

Fruits

The best fruits for PMS are those that are seasonal and grown in temperate climates. They tend to be higher in fiber and lower in sugar content. Fruits grown in the hot tropical sun tend to be much sweeter, which can worsen fluid retention and sugar craving in susceptible women.

Oils

Preferred oils include sesame oil, olive oil, corn oil, and safflower oil. Unlike animal fats, they are unsaturated. (All except olive oil are polyunsaturated.) Cold-pressed oils tend to be fresher and purer.

*Modified from Lark SM: The PMS Prevention Diet. New Woman February, 1985, p. 18

helps PMS is not clear, but in a preliminary observation[56] exercise was noted to increase β-EP levels, which may explain the sense of well-being reported by some patients. If β-EP withdrawal contributes to PMS, it might be corrected at least partially by exercise.

This general approach should be offered by a multidisciplinary team that integrates the efforts of a gynecologist, an endocrinologist, a psychiatrist or psychologist, a social worker, and a nutritionist, whether it is offered by a clinic within a university medical center or one that is free-standing. If no improvement is reported within 2 months using this approach, drug therapy aimed at target symptoms is added.

SPECIFIC APPROACH

Fluid Retention Symptoms

If the patient gains weight and experiences edema premenstrually, and weight loss occurs dramatically after the onset of menstruation, spironolactone 25 mg four times a day starting 10 days before the expected onset of menstruation is recommended. O'Brien et al.[57] have shown significant improvement in reduction in weight and psychological symptoms using spironolactone.

Breast Symptoms

The dopaminergic agonist bromocriptine 5 mg at night daily from days 10 to 26 of the cycle was noted to produce a significant reduction in breast tenderness and swelling[58] but was ineffective in controlling other symptoms of PMS. Danazol 200 mg twice daily also effectively suppressed breast symptoms.[59]

Headache and Other Pain

The prostaglandin synthetase inhibitor mefenamic acid blocks the production of prostaglandins and was found to ameliorate premenstrual symptoms in an uncontrolled study.[60,61] Mira et al.[62] in a double-blind, placebo-controlled study also showed that it significantly improved many symptoms, particularly fatigue, headache, general aches and pains, and mood swings. In that study, 15 PMS patients were investigated over six menstrual cycles; they were given 250 mg of mefenamic acid daily starting 12 days before the expected date of menses. Nonsteroidal anti-inflammatory agents such as acetylsalicylic acid or acetaminophen with or without codeine are also used to relieve headaches, musculoskeletal pain, and other pain syndromes.[47]

Somatic and Psychological Symptoms

If the patients have moderate to severe generalized symptoms, they require medication that can presumably correct the underlying pathophysiologic disorder. No one drug has been universally helpful for premenstrual changes, nor has the random, empiric approach been helpful.[63] Some patients do not respond to any treatment, and others respond to whatever they receive. Only a double-blind, crossover placebo-controlled clinical trial can demonstrate the efficacy of a treatment.

The role of psychological, environmental, and behavioral factors is illustrated by patients who continue having cyclic symptoms after natural or surgical menopause.[64] Although the severity of symptoms may decrease after hormone fluctuation ceases, symptoms persist. Hysterectomy is not indicated; bilateral oophorectomy might help but has not been evaluated and is rarely indicated unless there is coexisting pelvic pathology.[47]

A number of drugs have been used for PMS, e.g., oral contraceptives, progestens, diuretics, vitamin A, belladonna alkaloids, tranquilizers, lithium, antidepressants, and stimulants. Clinical trials have generally failed to demonstrate a consistent therapeutic effect.[6,63,65] Several research approaches are currently being utilized and can be divided into the following categories.

Clonidine   This antihypertensive agent has proved useful for the treatment of opiate withdrawal in addicts undergoing detoxification[66]; it may be anxiolytic. Its effect may be related to its activation of central α_2-adrenergic receptors. Nilsson et al.[67] reported relief of PMS symptoms in a patient given 25 µg of clonidine three times a day beginning 15 days before and ending 2 days after the start of menstruation. Slight sedation was the only side effect.[67]

Prince and Giannini[68] have described successful treatment with clonidine (17 µg/kg daily) in two women with premenstrual complaints. However, the dosage was much higher, and side effects, e.g., sedation and orthostatic hypotension, could be problematic. The efficacy of this therapy needs to be verified by large, controlled, double-blind trials.

Medical oophorectomy   In a crossover study conducted over a 6-month period, Muse et al.[69] demonstrated that elimination of ovarian cyclicity through down-regulation of pituitary gonadotropin secretion with a gonadotropin-releasing hormone (GnRH) agonist resulted in marked attenuation of premenstrual symptoms. Each of the eight patients received 50 µg of GnRH agonist daily by subcutaneous injection. The therapy was rapidly reversible, with no influence on subsequent cycles.[69] Bancroft et al.[70] showed similar results using buserelin, another GnRH agonist, in another study.

Depo-Medroxyprogesterone acetate (Depo-Provera), which is also used as a contraceptive, has also been used to treat PMS. Keye[71] reported a more than 50 percent reduction in the severity of PMS symptoms in 15 of 20 women who participated in an open clinical trial. Some of the women noted that the duration of the effect of the drug was only 4 weeks despite the fact that the anovulatory effect lasted at least 3 months. Danazol has been shown to be effective only for the control of breast symptoms[59]; however, more studies on its relation to other PMS symptoms are currently being conducted.

Medical oophorectomy may prevent the fluctuation of β-EP levels by causing temporary cessation of cyclic ovarian activity. Unfortunately, the efficacy of these drugs is problematic, as patients are amenorrheic while taking medication, and the safety of long-term therapy remains to be determined.

Progesterone   Dalton's original study reported complete relief of symptoms in more than 83 percent of a group of 86 PMS women.[72] Although others question its efficacy, progesterone administration has remained popular. It has been used as a vaginal suppository, a buccal tablet, a capsule, a dermal patch, a rectal suppository/spray, a suspension, and a gel. However, several studies have shown that progesterone vaginal suppository is not superior to placebo in double-blind, controlled clinical trials[73-76] despite higher circulating progesterone levels found with this route of administration.[76,77] In contrast, another study[78] showed that orally administered micronized progesterone benefits patients with PMS in a double-blind, placebo-controlled, 4-month trial. Each of the 23 patients were given one 100-mg capsule in the morning and two 100-mg capsules at night for 10 days of each cycle starting 3 days after ovulation. Problems with this study include only one-month pretreatment assessment, and no changes in plasma gonadotropins, prolactin, progesterone, or estradiol before treatment. However, estrogen and progesterone have been noted to increase β-EP levels in portal blood samples collected from ovariectomized monkeys,[79] which suggests that the beneficial effect of progesterone may be mediated by β-EP.

Vitamin B$_6$ Estrogen-induced deficiency in vitamin B$_6$ leading to serotonin deficiency has been postulated to cause depression in oral contraceptive users,[80] and significant improvement following vitamin B$_6$ therapy has been reported.[81] To date, the clinical response to vitamin B$_6$ in PMS patients has not been adequately evaluated. Vitamin B$_6$ deficiency has not been demonstrated in patients compared to controls.

In an ongoing study we measure peripheral levels of vitamin B$_6$ in affected women and controls. Several patients have shown a decrease in vitamin B$_6$ during the luteal phase compared with the follicular phase; some showed no change, and some showed an increase. Controls showed either an increase or no change during the luteal phase; none showed a decrease. Taylor et al. also reported that some PMS patients had less than 50 percent RDA for vitamin B$_6$ and 68 to 84 percent RDA for magnesium in their nutrient intakes. Less severe symptoms of PMS were reported after vitamin B$_6$ treatment[82]; however the vitamin B$_6$ levels were not assessed before or after treatment. A premenstrual decrease in vitamin B$_6$ levels could identify a subgroup of PMS patients in whom vitamin B$_6$ deficiency plays a role and who may respond to vitamin B$_6$ therapy.

The daily requirement for vitamin B$_6$ is 2 to 4 mg, and a daily dose of 50 to 300 mg has been suggested for treatment of PMS. However, peripheral neuropathy has been reported with vitamin B$_6$ administration of 200 to 6,000 mg daily.[83] Abraham has reported tolerance to vitamin B$_6$ within 6 months where vitamin B$_6$ requirements are increased when it is given without other supplements.[39] He recommended megadoses of vitamin B$_6$ with other micronutrients to minimize the side effects of vitamin B$_6$. For example, both magnesium and riboflavin are required for the conversion of pyridoxine, the form of vitamin B$_6$ used in supplement, which is inactive to the active form. He proposed a combination of vitamin B$_6$ and other essential micronutrients for use in the management of PMS and showed that it reduced the severity of symptoms at daily doses of 2 to 12 tablets that contained 100 to 600 mg of vitamin B$_6$.[39] Further evaluation of this therapy is needed.

Naltrexone   The β-EP withdrawal hypothesis suggests treatment of PMS with exogenous β-EP, but it is not practical because of addiction and the route of administration (intramuscular or intravenous). An opiate antagonist, given before the periovulatory β-EP peak and withdrawal might offer a rational treatment for PMS by keeping a rather constant level of β-EP. Naltrexone is an oral pure narcotic antagonist that has been used in the treatment of withdrawal symptoms for patients with heroin addiction. Unlike drugs that have mixed agonist and antagonist effects, it does not cause addiction or withdrawal.[84]

We conducted the following double-blind, crossover, placebo-controlled study.[85] Twenty women with the diagnosis of PMS seen at the Mayo Clinic received either placebo or naltrexone 25 mg twice daily on days 9 to 18 of the menstrual cycle for three consecutive cycles. The dosage of 25 mg bid was chosen as 50 mg daily has been found to block the effects of heroin[84] and presumably of endogenous opiates as well. The preovulatory onset schedule was designed to inhibit opiate withdrawal. Sixteen patients completed the study. The mean of three day-25 Menstrual Distress Questionnaire scores of the 16 patients revealed that for 11 patients the score was at least 10 points lower on naltrexone, the scores of 2 patients increased at least 10 points, and 3 patients had changes of less than 10 points. The mean scores dropped 28 points on naltrexone ($p = 0.016$), and there was no evidence of a carry-over effect with naltrexone. These results suggest that naltrexone alleviates PMS symptoms and may be an effective treatment for this syndrome. Further studies in this area are currently being conducted. The side effects of naltrexone reported in the literature include nausea, abdominal pain, headache, and skin rash; however, the incidence is low, and it is considered to be a safe medication.[86] The acceptability of this medication in our study was good despite some incidence of nausea, decreased appetite, and dizziness/fainting, which may be minimized by further dividing or decreasing the dosage.

FUTURE CONSIDERATIONS

There are several areas in which additional research efforts are needed:

1. The development of a standard, universally accepted questionnaire/assessment tool to diagnose and evaluate the severity of symptoms is needed. At present, various clinician/researcher groups use different questionnaires, and it is difficult to compare results from different centers.

2. A biochemical marker to help with diagnosis and evaluation of treatment is needed.

3. Classification of PMS into subgroups is needed. It might be based on the predominant and initial presentation of somatic and psychological symptoms, and their timing in reference to the menstrual cycle, as well as laboratory findings, e.g., hormone or vitamin levels. This classification scheme can help identify characteristics of each subgroup and predict successful treatment response.

4. The pathophysiology needs to be investigated. Effective treatment for PMS does not exist due in part to the fact that the physiology of mood and behavior is not well understood. Investigations in this area are certainly needed.

It is possible that PMS results from an aberration of normal cycle changes in β-EP or the activity of other neurotransmitters during the luteal phase. Research is needed to establish the temporal relation between cyclic symptoms and endocrine changes and to identify endocrine factors that may be relevant to PMS. Ultimately, treatment should address the underlying pathophysiologic mechanisms, and evaluation of treatment should rely on biologic measures (e.g., hormone levels) in addition to clinical observation.

ACKNOWLEDGMENT

We acknowledge with appreciation Ms. Lynne C. Matous for her excellent editorial assistance during the preparation of this chapter.

REFERENCES

1. Frank RT: The hormonal causes of premenstrual tension. Arch Neurol Psychiatry 26:1053, 1931
2. Shabanah EH: Treatment of premenstrual tension. Obstet Gynecol 21:49, 1963
3. Dalton K: The influence of menstruation on health and disease. Proc R Soc Med 57:262, 1964
4. Dalton K: Menstruation and crime. Br Med J 2:1752, 1961
5. Bicker W, Woods M: Premenstrual tension-rational treatment. Tex Rep Biol Med 9:406, 1951
6. Reid RL, Yen SSC: Premenstrual syndrome. Am J Obstet Gynecol 139:85, 1981
7. Watts JF, Butt WR, Edwards RL: Hormonal studies in women with premenstrual tension. Br J Obstet Gynaecol 92:247, 1985
8. Sondheimer SJ, Freeman EW, Scharlop B, et al: Hormonal changes in premenstrual syndrome. Psychosomatics 26:803, 1985
9. Munday MR, Brush MG, Taylor RW: Correlates between progesterone, oestradiol and aldosterone levels in the premenstrual syndrome. Clin Endocrinol (Oxf) 14:1, 1981
10. Steiner M, Haskett RF, Carroll BJ: Circadian hormone secretory profiles in women with severe premenstrual tension syndrome. Br J Obstet Gynaecol 91:466, 1984
11. Backstrom T, Mattsson B: Correlation of symptoms in premenstrual tension in oestrogen and progesterone concentrations in blood plasma. Neuropsychobiology 1:80, 1975
12. Andersch B, Abrahamsson L, Wendestem C, et al: Hormone profiles in premenstrual tension: effects of bromocriptine and diurectics. Clin Endocrinol (Oxf) 11:657, 1979
13. Butt WR, Watt JF, Holder G: The biochemical background to the premenstrual syndrome. p. 16. In Taylor RW (ed): Premenstrual Syndrome. Medical New-Tribune, London, 1983
14. Backstrom T, Wide L, Sodergard R, et al: FSH, LH, TeBG capacity, estrogen and progesterone in women with premenstrual tension during the luteal phase. J Steroid Biochem 7:473, 1976
15. Dalton M: Sex hormone-binding globulin concentrations in women with severe premenstrual syndrome. Postgrad Med J 57:560, 1981
16. Charvat J, Holececk V: Studies on antidiuretic hormone. Acta Med Acad Sci Hung 23:81, 1966

17. Carroll BJ: The dexamethasone suppression test for melancholia. Br J Psychiatry 140:292, 1982
18. Muse K, Vernon M, Wilson E: Decreased dexamethasone suppression of cortisol in premenstrual syndrome. p. 93. In: Society for Gynecologic Investigation 33rd Annual Meeting Abstracts, 1986
19. Reid RL: Premenstrual syndrome. Curr Probl Obstet Gynecol Fertil 8(2):3, 1985
20. Chuong CJ, Colligan CR, Coulam CB, et al: The Minnesota Multiphasic Personality Inventory (MMPI) as an aid in evaluating the patients with premenstrual syndrome. Presented at the 34th Annual Clinical Meeting of the American College of Obstetricians and Gynecologists, New Orleans, 1986
21. Keye WR, Hammond DC, Strong T: Medical and psychologic characteristics of women presenting with premenstrual symptoms. Obstet Gynecol 68:635, 1986
22. Friedman R, et al: Sexual histories and premenstrual affective syndrome in psychiatric in-patients. Am Psychiatry 39:1484, 1982
23. Harrison WM, Rabkin JG, Endicott J: Psychiatric evaluation of premenstrual changes. Psychosomatics 26:789, 1985
24. Thorn GW, Nelson KR, Thorn DW: Study of the mechanism of oedema associated with menstruation. Endocrinology 22:155, 1938
25. O'Brien PMS, Selby C, Symonds EM: Progesterone, fluid and electrolytes in premenstrual syndrome. Br Med J 280:1161, 1980
26. Bruce J, Russell GPM: Premenstrual tension: a study of weight changes and balances of water, sodium and potassium. Lancet 2:267, 1962
27. Davidson BJ, Valenzuela GJ: Atrial natriuretic factor and plasma renin activity in women with premenstrual syndrome, sex steroid therapy and pregnancy. p. 114. In: American Fertility Society 42nd Annual Meeting Abstracts, 1986
28. Klein L, Carey J: Total exchangeable sodium in the menstrual cycle. Am J Obstet Gynecol 74:956, 1957
29. Jordan, VC, Pokoly TB: Steroid and prostaglandin relations during the menstrual cycle. Obstet Gynecol 49:449, 1977
30. Jakubowicz DL: The significance of prostaglandins in the premenstrual syndrome. p. 50. In Taylor RW (ed): Premenstrual Syndrome. Medical New-Tribune, London, 1983
31. Morton JH, Additon H, Addison RG, et al: A clinical study of premenstrual tension. Am J Obstet Gynecol 65:1182, 1953
32. Reid RL, Greenaway-Coates A, Hahn PM: Menstrual cycle related changes in glucose, insulin and glucagon following an oral glucose load in normal women and in women with premenstrual "hypoglycemic attacks." p. 194. In: Society of Gynecologic Investigation 32nd Annual Meeting Abstracts, 1985
33. Reid RL, Greenaway-Coates A, Hahn PM: Oral glucose tolerance during the menstrual cycle in normal women and women with alleged premenstrual "hypoglycemic" attacks: Effects of nalozone. J Clin Endocrinol Metab 62:1167, 1986
34. Israel SL: Premenstrual tension. JAMA 110:1721, 1938
35. Morton JH: Premenstrual tension. Am J Obstet Gynecol 60:343, 1950
36. Biskind MS, Biskind GR: Inactivation of testosterone propionate in the liver during vitamin B complex deficiency: alteration of the estrogen-androgen equilibrium. Endocrinology 32:97, 1943
37. Zondek B, Brezezinski A: Inactivation of oestrogenic hormone by women with vitamin B deficiency. Br J Obstet Gynaecol 55:273, 1948
38. Asberg M: Chemical factor found among causes of suicide. NY Acad Sci 1:1, 1986

39. Abraham GE: Management of the premenstrual tension syndromes: rationale for a nutritional approach, p. 144. In Bland J (ed): A Year in Nutritional Medicine: 1986. Keates, New Caanan, CT, 1986.

40. Volavka J, Davis LG, Ehrlich YH: Endorphins, dopamine and schizophrenia. Schizophr Bull 5:227, 1979

41. Wehrenberg WB, Waralaw SL, Franz AG, et al: β-Endorphin in hypophyseal portal blood: variations throughout the menstrual cycle. Endocrinology 111:879, 1982

42. Wardlaw SL, Wehrenberg WB, Ferin M, et al: Effects of sex steroids on β-endorphin in hypophyseal portal blood. J Clin Endocrinol Metab 55:877, 1982

43. Gintzler D: Endorphin-mediated increases in pain during pregnancy. Science 210:193, 1980

44. Lindstrom LH, Widerlov E, Gunne LM, et al: Endorphins in human cerebrospinal fluid: clinical correlations to some psychotic states. Acta Psychiatr Scand 57:153, 1978

45. Cohen MR, Cohen, RM, Pecker D, et al: Behavior effects after high dose naloxone administration to normal volunteers. Lancet 2:1110, 1981

46. Reid RL, Greenaway-Coats A, Hahn PM, et al: Menopausal-like hot flashes in women of reproductive age: a clue to the pathophysiology of premenstrual syndrome. p. 194. In: American Fertility Society 42nd Annual Meeting Abstracts, 1986

47. Reid RL, Yen SSC: The premenstrual syndrome. Clin Obstet Gynecol 26:710, 1983

48. Quigley ME, Yen SSC: The role of endogenous opiates on LH secretions during the menstrual cycle. J Clin Endocrinol Metab 51:179, 1980

49. Vargyas JM, Lobo RA, Mishell D: Brain opioid activity in the premenstrual syndrome. Presented at the 33rd Annual Clinical Meeting of the American College of Obstetricians and Gynecologists, Washington, DC, 1985.

50. Chuong CJ, Coulam CB, Kao PC, et al: Neuropeptide levels in premenstrual syndrome. Fertil Steril 44:760, 1985

51. Jeffcoate WJ, Reese LH, McLoughlin L, et al: β-Endorphin in human cerebrospinal fluid. Lancet 2:119, 1978

52. Margules DL, Moisset B, Lewis MJ, et al: β-Endorphins in association with overeating in genetically obese mice (ob/ob) and rats (la/la). Science 202:988, 1978

53. Moos RH: The development of a menstrual distress questionnaire. Psychosom Med 30:853, 1968

54. Steiner M, Haskett RF, Carroll BJ: Premenstrual tension syndrome: the development of research diagnosis criteria and new rating scales. Acta Psychiatr Scand 62:177, 1980

54a. Lark SM: The PMS Prevention Diet. New Woman February 1985, p. 18.

55. Timonen S, Procope BJ: Premenstrual syndrome and physical exercise. Acta Obstet Gynecol Scand 50:331, 1971

56. Carr DB, Buller BA, Skrinar GS et al: Physical conditioning facilitates the exercise-induced secretion of beta endorphin and beta-lipotropin in women. N Engl J Med 305:560, 1981

57. O'Brien PMS, Craven D, Selby C, et al: Treatment of premenstrual syndrome by spironolactone. Br J Obstet Gynaecol 86:142, 1979

58. Mansel RE, Wisbey JR, Hughes LE: The use of danazol in the treatment of painful benign breast disease: preliminary results. Postgrad Med J, suppl. 5, 55:51, 1979

59. Day J: Danzol and the premenstrual syndrome. Postgrad Med J 55:87, 1979

60. Wood C, Jakubowicz DL: The treatment of premenstrual tension with mefenamic acid. Br J Obstet Gynaecol 87:627, 1980

61. Jakubowicz DL, Dewhurst J: The treatment of premenstrual tension and mefena-

mic acid: analysis of prostaglandin concentrations. Br J Obstet Gynaecol 91:78, 1984

62. Mira M, McNeil D, Fraser IS, et al: Mefenamic acid in the treatment of premenstrual syndrome. Obstet Gynecol 68:395, 1986

63. O'Brien PMS: The premenstrual syndrome. J Reprod Med 30:113, 1985

64. Dalton K: The Premenstrual Syndrome and Progesterone Therapy. Heinemann, London, 1984

65. DeVane GW, Lasley BL: Efficacy of amphetamine treatment for severe premenstrual syndrome. p. 86. In: American Fertility Society 42nd Annual Meeting Abstracts, 1986

66. Gold MS, Kleber HD: Clinical utility of clonidine in opiate withdrawal: a study of 100 patients. p. 299. In Lal H, Fieding S (eds): Psychopharmacology of Clonidine. Alan R. Liss, New York, 1981

67. Nilsson LC, Ericksson E, Carlsson M, et al: Clonidine for relief of premenstrual syndrome. Lancet 2:549, 1985

68. Price WA, Giannini AJ: The use of clonidine in premenstrual tension syndrome. J Clin Pharmacol 24:463, 1984

69. Muse KN, Cetel NS, Futterman LA, et al: The premenstrual syndrome: effects of "medical ovariectomy." N Engl J Med 311:1345, 1984

70. Bancroft J, Boyle H, Davidson DW, et al: The effects of an LHRH agonist on the premenstrual syndrome: a preliminary report. In: Proceedings of International Workshop on LHRH and Its Analogues: Fertility and Antifertility Aspects, Berlin, 1984

71. Keye WR: Depomedroxyprogesterone acetate in premenstrual syndrome. Presented at the First International Symposium on Premenstrual Syndrome and Dysmenorrhea, Kiawah Island, SC, 1983

72. Greene R, Dalton K: Premenstrual syndrome. Br Med J 1:1007, 1953

73. Smith SL: Mood and the menstrual cycle. In: Sacher EJ (ed): Topics in Psychoendrocrinology. Grune & Stratton, New York, 1975

74. Sampson G: Premenstrual syndrome: a double-blind controlled trial of progesterone and placebo. Br J Psychiatry 135:209, 1979

75. Maddocks SG, Hahn PM, Moller F, et al: A double blind placebo-controlled trial of progresterone vaginal suppositories in the treatment of premenstrual syndrome. Am J Obstet Gynecol 154:573, 1986

76. Vargyas JM, Marrs RP: The use of progesterone in the premenstrual syndrome. p. 1. In: American Fertility Society 41st Annual Meeting Abstracts, 1985

77. Myers ER, Sondheimer SJ, Freeman EW, et al: Serum progresterone levels after vaginal administration during the luteal phase in premenstrual syndrome patients. p. 76. In: American Fertility Society 41st Annual Meeting Abstracts, 1985

78. Dennerstein L, Spencer-Gardner C, Gotts G, et al: Progesterone and the premenstrual syndrome: a double blind crossover trial. Br Med J 290:1617, 1985

79. Wardlaw SL, Wehrenberg WB, Ferin M, et al: Effect of sex steroids on β-endophin in hypophyseal portal blood. J Clin Endocrinol Metab 55:877, 1982

80. Rose DP: The interactions between vitamin B_6 and hormones. Vitam Horm 36:53, 1978

81. Adams PW, Rose DP, Folkard J, et al: Effect of pyridoxine hydochloride (vitamin B_6) upon depression associated with oral contraception. Lancet 1:897, 1973

82. Taylor ML, Krutan MS, Freeman E: Vitamin B_6 status of women with premenstrual syndrome. Fed Proc 44:776, 1985

83. Parr GJ, Brodesen DE: Sensory neuropathy with low dose pyridoxine. Neurology 35:1466, 1985.

84. Renault PF: Treatment of heroin-dependent persons with antagonists: current status. p. 11. In Willette RE, Barnett G (eds): Naltrexone Research Monograph 28. National Institute on Drug Abuse, Washington, DC, 1980

85. Chuong CJ, Coulam CB, Bergstralh EJ, et al: Clinical trial of naltrexone in premenstrual syndrome. In: 34th American College of Obstetricians and Gynecologists District VII Meeting Abstracts, section 2B, 1986

86. O'Brien CP, Greenstein RG, Mintz J, et al: Clinical experience with naltrexone. Am J Drug Alcohol Abuse 2:365, 1975

8

Clinical Evaluation
and Management

Howard J. Osofsky
William Henry Keppel

Since the initial description of premenstrual tension by Frank in 1931,[1] a number of etiologic explanations, evaluation protocols, and strategies for treatment have been offered in an attempt to understand and alleviate premenstrual symptoms. Contributing to the discouragement of clinicians and researchers, most of the hypotheses and treatment regimens have not stood the test of time. In general, studies have been poorly designed; patient selection has been confounded by nonverified retrospective data and questionable inclusion criteria; placebo-controlled, double-blind crossover studies have not been carried out; follow-up has been inadequate; and results have not been replicated. Mechanisms of hormonal interaction have been proposed, but endocrine assays, when performed, have frequently not been timed appropriately, have been insufficient in number, and have relied on questionable laboratory techniques. Furthermore, given the state of the art, they have often been indirect and reflective of peripheral, rather than target, levels of the substances assessed. Evaluation and treatment strategies have often been based on questionable theoretical frameworks. It is of some encouragement that serious attempts have begun to be made to provide scientifically sound evaluation and management efforts. At present these efforts remain in the early stages, and they are not sufficient to provide clear clinical directions.

In this chapter we consider clinical approaches to the evaluation and treatment of premenstrual symptoms. We emphasize at this point, as we do throughout the chapter, that the treatment regimens described, although frequently employed, in general have not been verified by replicated double-blind placebo-controlled crossover studies. However, because a number of them are in wide use at this time, it seems worthwhile to try to understand the rationale for such approaches and some of the clinical considerations in their use. We recognize that further theoretically and methodologically sound studies are needed, and that when they are carried out they will likely influence and change evaluation and treatment strategies.

DEFINITIONS AND PATTERNS OF SYMPTOMS

The first step in evaluation is clarity as to what is being evaluated. Our definition of premenstrual syndromes, which agrees with that of other workers in this field, states that the symptoms must have a cyclic, recurrent component that is related to the menstrual cycle. There is generally an interval, either free of symptoms or with marked improvement, usually during the follicular phase of the cycle with an exacerbation and worsening of symptoms usually occurring premenstrually.

Estimates indicate that most women have some premenstrual symptoms; in various reports the range is between 20 and 90 percent, and 3 to 15 percent have severe symptoms. Women have a variety of symptom complexes with different implications; as a result, we prefer the term *premenstrual syndromes* to *premenstrual syndrome* for PMS.

Rubinow and Roy-Byrne[2] listed a number of the common symptoms of premenstrual syndromes. They described affective, cognitive, painful, neurovegetative, autonomic, central nervous system, fluid/electrolyte, dermatologic, and behavioral symptoms. Perhaps in a somewhat more simplified framework, one can divide the symptoms into those of a physical nature and those of an emotional nature. Obviously there is considerable overlap. Under such a schema, physical symptoms include the following: those of an allergic nature; gastrointestinal symptoms including food cravings, constipation, and diarrhea; low abdominal and pelvic discomfort and bloating; joint and muscle discomfort and stiffness; pain and swelling in the breasts; and a variety of nervous system complaints such as headache, clumsiness, difficulties with concentration and memory, and seizures. Emotional symptoms include the following: mood swings; irritability; anxiety, depression, sometimes with suicidal ideations; difficulties with control, at times including violence; eating patterns suggestive of bulimia; and psychoses. Patients may report increases or decreases in levels of energy and sexual desire; outbursts and fluctuations of symptoms may provide further confusion and distress for the patient.

In addition, premenstrual syndromes are generally described as agerelated, with symptoms usually increasing during the late twenties, thirties, and forties. Symptoms occurring early in adolescence have been correlated with earlier onset of menarche; but as with older patients, there is no clear relation to regularity of the menstrual cycle. In young women the symptoms do not appear to be clearly related to those of their mothers but are related to lack of preparation for menstrration and to the mother's expectations of her symptoms.

There appear to be links between emotional symptoms that are related to the menstrual cycle and emotional symptoms related to other important events in the female reproductive life cycle, e.g., postpartum depression, depression after perinatal loss, oral contraceptive-related depression, and menopausal depression. In our experience, a number of patients report a worsening of symptoms during the first several months to 1 year following tubal ligation. Symptoms have also been reported after hysterectomy, with and without bilateral oophorectomy. Of course, it should be noted that premenstrual symptoms and dysmenorrhea are currently seen by obstetricians and gynecologists as separate symptoms. In high quality gynecologically oriented evaluation programs, significant percentages of patients with severe symptoms appear to have emotional components to their symptoms; the corollary is also true that patients with predominantly emotional symptoms may have physical or physiologically determined components to their symptoms.

ETIOLOGY

A number of theories have been put forth to explain the etiology of premenstrual syndromes. Other chapters in this volume deal with this area in depth. Therefore although it is an important topic, we do not attempt to deal with it in this chapter.

EVALUATION

PROSPECTIVE RATINGS

As emphasized by others, we also stress that the first, and perhaps most important, step in the management with patients with premenstrual symptoms is a careful evaluation. When possible, we believe that it is important to obtain a careful initial history and then prospectively follow the patient's symptoms for 3 months prior to instituting treatment per se. Table 8-1 is a list of symptoms that we ask patients to rate in terms of severity on a daily basis; other symptoms of concern to specific individuals are included as indicated. In addition, the patients record information related to daily stresses, ovulation, and menstruation. We also utilize the visual analogue scales developed by Rubinow, and symptom, personal, family, and medical history forms that are being used in a number of other centers.

It seems important to emphasize the value of the 3 months of prospective ratings. In our experience, as well as that of others, approximately 50 percent of the patients either drop out or require no further treatment by the end of this time interval. After preliminary discussions and initial general advice, some women describe learning self-treatment techniques as they chart their symptoms and the factors that appear to trigger the worsening of symptoms. For example, women may come to sense that although they at times crave sweets, caffeine, cigarettes, and/or alcohol symptoms worsen following their use. Some learn that exercise on a regular basis appears to decrease their symptoms. Women may become aware of triggering factors and events in their lives and develop scheduling techniques and other methods of dealing with situational factors that help alleviate the symptoms. Some women find that they bring things under better control owing to their newly found pre-

TABLE 8-1. SYMPTOMS ROUTINELY CHARTED
Angry/irritable
Cramps
Crying/feeling like crying
Depressed
Disturbing thoughts
Empty feeling
Energy decreased, sleepiness, fatigue, lethargy, social isolation
Energy increased, agitation
Fat feeling, bloating
Food cravings, anorexia
Hallucinations
Headaches; other pain; breast, joint, and muscle symptoms
Nervous
Out of control, poor impulse control
Sexual interest—increased
Sexual interest—decreased
Suicidal
Unreal feeling
Violent feeling
Weights recorded daily
Basal body temperatures taken daily

Other symptoms
  Anxiety symptoms, tension, nausea, diarrhea, palpitations, sweating
  Neurologic symptoms
  Dermatologic symptoms
  Allergic symptoms

dictabilities from charting and no longer feel the need for further work-up. It has been our sense that, for a number of the women, having professionals who are available and caring and who acknowledge the legitimacy of their symptoms serves to diminish the urgency of the symptoms and allows for improved self-care techniques of coping with them. Thus a group of patients exist who can learn to productively accept and live with their symptoms; thus the prospective symptom study period itself has a therapeutic effect.

Of the remaining women, at the end of the 3-month interval we have noted a number of patterns. About one-half of the women appear to have significant symptoms but with the symptoms apparently unrelated to the menstrual cycle. This figure generally agrees with studies of others. Such women may benefit from further psychiatric or medical evaluation and treatment. Of the remaining women, a number of pictures have emerged, and we are currently questioning the meaning of these symptoms.

SYMPTOMS RELATED TO
THE MENSTRUAL CYCLE

For those women who have significant symptoms related to the menstrual cycle, our work-up consists of the following evaluations that are scheduled at the height of symptoms, with repeat evaluations taking place as indicated during a symptom-free interval.

1. *General assessments.* Perhaps it goes without saying that we take a careful history of the symptoms, their duration, and precipitating factors; associated psychiatric symptoms, including typical and atypical vegetative components; alcohol and drug use patterns; prior treatment approaches and outcome; and a family history, including a review of family relationships, menstrual difficulties, and psychiatric (especially affective) disorders.
2. *Medical evaluation.* It includes a full medical history and physical examination, including a pelvic examination. Special emphasis is placed on possible endocrine, metabolic, neurologic, and gynecologic disorders.
3. *Nutritional assessment.* It includes typical daily dietary patterns, with additional emphasis on areas of deficiency and other abnormalities that might be expected to relate to premenstrual symptoms.
4. *Laboratory tests.* They include a complete blood count, blood chemistry profile, urinalysis, blood sugars, T_3, T_4, thyrotropin-releasing hormone (TRH) stimulation test, dexamethasone suppression test, vitamin B_6 and magnesium levels, extradiol, progesterone, and prolactin levels, Papanicolaou smear with assessment for hormonal status, and, depending on neurologic and cognitive symptoms, electroencephalography (EEG) and neurometric assessments.
5. *Psychological testing.* Related to our setting, we administer a standard battery of psychological tests, including a TAT, Rorschach, and WAIS, and other assessments as indicated. This protocol obviously is not feasible or appropriate for all clinical facilities.

SOME OVERALL FINDINGS

Consistent with Brook-Gunn and Ruble's data (personal communication, 1984), we have noted a greater relation between the patient's symptoms and her mother's attitudes and other background characteristics than between the patient's and her mother's symptoms. A variety of diagnosed gynecologic difficulties have been linked with physical symptoms. Menstrual irregularity has been accompanied or influenced by emotional symptoms. A number of patients, especially those with significant symptoms that either appear sporadically or are present throughout the menstrual cycle, have demonstrated underlying psychiatric difficulty. On psychological testing, especially prominent has been an increase in dependency needs, perhaps related to the improvement in symptoms when the patients enter a therapeutic relationship. We have now seen four patients in whom EEG or neurometric patterns have evidenced differences related to the menstrual cycle. It is of some note that the differences corresponded to such patient symptoms as seizures, clumsiness, difficulty concentrating, parasthesias, or other possibly neurologically based complaints. This finding is consistent with the reports of catamenial epilepsy noted in the literature and described by Newmark and Penrey.[3] To date, we have been disappointed in the findings from the dexamethasone suppression tests, the TRH stimulation tests, and in general the estradiol and progesterone determinations. We are currently considering obtaining dexamethasone suppression tests and the possibility of different hormonal assessments.

TREATMENT

The focus here is on hormonal and other medical approaches to treatment, rather than the role of psychotropic medications. We approach this section with some trepidation because of the lack of methodologically sound placebo-controlled crossover studies. Medications are currently being prescribed with questionable theoretical rationale and without confirmatory data related to absorption patterns, outcome, or follow-up. Other medications are being prescribed without Food and Drug Administration (FDA) approval. Yet we are respectful of the fact that good clinicians have the sense that some medications are of benefit at least in some cases.

It seems important to emphasize that at this time, with the fragmentary knowledge at hand, there is no one answer or no right answer. No single treatment regimen has been proved effective for a specific group or groups of PMS patients. We therefore advise clinicians to be cautious if they are prescribing medications, to use approaches that appear to be pharmacologically safest, and to leave more experimental approaches for last. Most good programs do not promise patients a cure but inform them that they try to help alleviate the symptoms. We encourage clinicians to follow patients carefully, to look for side effects, to be open to the possibility of failure, and to assess the need for alternate approaches. A number of programs have noted that, among some women whose symptoms are alleviated, after an initial period of improvement there may be a return of symptoms or the appearance of new symptoms. We have had patients referred to us who have been treated with various regimens and who have had persistent or recurrent symptoms but have been afraid to discuss these symptoms with their treaters because of their sense of the treaters' enthusiasm for a given therapeutic regimen. Lack of knowledge about just such cases is likely to influence adversely clinicians' approaches to treatment.

With this in mind, we summarize some current approaches that are commonly utilized for treatment. Again, we emphasize that methodologically sound data are not present to substantiate clearly the efficacy of various treatment regimens, and that with further research studies better theoretical and clinical understanding may be possible in the coming years.[2] Yet we recognize that many women are currently requesting treatment for symptoms re-

TABLE 8-2. TREATMENT OF PREMENSTRUAL SYMPTOMS

Contact with professionals who are empathetic, informed, and available

Modifications in diet (sugar, white flour, caffeine, chocolate)

Decreased or discontiued alcohol consumption

Decreased or discontinued smoking

Exercise

Stress reduction or psychotherapy

Vitamins (vitamin B_6)

Minerals (magnesium)

Hormones (progesterones, oral contraceptive steroids)

Diuretics (spironolactone)

Bromocriptine

Danazol

Antiprostaglandins

lated to the menstrual cycle and that clinicians are prescribing it. For that reason, we discuss some current treatment approaches, with the provisions noted above (Table 8-2).

INITIAL GENERAL APPROACHES

Whenever possible we begin with a regimen that incorporates exercise, a well-balanced diet including decreased intake of refined sugars, white flour, coffee, tea, and chocolate, and decreased alcohol consumption prior to and during the time of the symptoms. We encourage women to decrease or discontinue smoking. There is a logical rationale to encouraging regular exercise in that exercise appears to affect endorphin balance,[4] and endorphins have been postulated as playing an etiologic role in PMS.[5] Although hypoglycemic patterns have not been demonstrated in association with PMS per se, based on studies of endocrinologically related varying glucose utilization the dietary recommendations also have some rationale.[6] If possible, we attempt to help women to identify and control stressors that appear to trigger symptoms. Recognizing the biasing factors in the types of women who are referred to us, in our experience a number of women appear to benefit substantially from individual psychotherapy and/or family therapy.

VITAMINS

For women whose dietary picture or whose laboratory testing indicates the appropriateness, multiple vitamins with at times the addition of pyridoxine or magnesium are prescribed. Those who support the use of pyridoxine suggest that it may be reduced in competitive inhibition by estrogen, may enhance estrogen clearance, and may augment biosynthesis of brain monoamines.[5,7] In uncontrolled studies there have been suggestive beneficial effects of both pyridoxine and magnesium. However, it seems important to emphasize that even such apparently innocuous treatments may not be free of side effects. In one study the use of 2,000 to 6,000 mg of pyridoxine daily resulted in signs of peripheral neuropathy,[8] and even 400 mg daily has been questioned as being hazardous to some individuals.[9] These symptoms gradually improved when the pyridoxine supplementation was discontinued. When utilized for premenstrual symptoms, pyridoxine and magnesium have most commonly been prescribed in doses of 100 to 300 mg daily; the dose of pyridoxine should certainly be kept well below 2,000 mg daily.

PROGESTERONE

Natural progesterone given by rectal suspension or vaginal or rectal suppository has had numerous proponents in the United States and elsewhere. It has been most popularized by the work of Dalton[10] in England, who claimed to substantiate its benefits in large numbers of patients under a wide variety of circumstances. The theoretical rationale has rested on a relative progesterone deficiency or estrogen excess. To date, such hormonal imbalances have not been substantiated. It remains possible that the pharmacologic doses utilized could have some unknown central nervous system effects that would relate to the amelioration of premenstrual symptoms; however, this area needs further investigation. The two studies that have utilized progesterone in a double-blind design, suffering from their own methodologic problems, failed to substantiate the efficacy of progesterone treatment.[11,12] It remains a widely utilized approach at the present time, however, and a number of clinicians believe that it has a useful role, at least for selected patients.

The usual starting dose of progesterone is 25 to 100 mg intramuscularly every other day or 200 to 400 mg daily by vaginal or rectal suppository from midcycle until the onset of menstruation; some physicians discontinue the progesterone 1 to 2 days prior to expected menstruation. If the dose does not control the symptoms, or if after a period of initial control the symptoms return, increasing amounts of progesterone have been applied, usually up to 1,600 mg daily by suppository. To date, reported side effects have been relatively minor. Patients may experience sedation, dysphoria, or worsening of depressive symptoms, especially when they have been a prominent component of the difficulty, and a possible worsening of vaginal candidiasis. However, although no long-term difficulties have been substantiated, concern has been raised about possible long-term metabolic, cardiovascular, and neoplastic side effects in patients or subsequent generations. Moreover, progesterone is known to be an immunosuppressant. Because of the sedating qualities of progesterone, some have recommended it primarily for patients with symptoms of anxiety, irritability, or volatility. Similarly, because of side effects of depression, if it is used at all it should be used with caution or in lower doses in women who have primary symptoms of severe depression,[13] especially if suicidal features are prominent. It should also be emphasized that patients with primary underlying psychiatric disorders with premenstrual exacerbation of symptoms should undergo evaluation and appropriate treatment for the underlying psychiatric difficulty. Progesterone is not contraindicated in women with seizure disorders and indeed raises the threshold of seizures. Progesterone is not an effective contraceptive. Because of a possible low incidence of fetal disorders, progesterone should not be started in a cycle where unprotected intercourse has taken place, and women taking progesterone are counseled to use appropriate contraception.

Medroxyprogesterone acetate tablets (Provera) and oral contraceptive steroids have also been used to treat premenstrual symptoms. Both regimens have the advantage of greater ease of administration and lesser cost compared to progesterone. As with progesterone, double-blind studies have not been performed that substantiate the efficacy of these statements. Of the studies that are available related to the use of medroxyprogesterone, both improvement and worsening of symptoms, as well as no differential effects from placebo have been reported. If medroxyprogesterone acetate tablets are utilized, the usual dose is 10 to 20 mg daily beginning on day 14 of the cycle, and being either discontinued at menstruation or tapered on the days prior to anticipated menstruation.

As with medroxyprogesterone acetate, some women report dramatic improvement of premenstrual symptoms while taking oral contraceptive steroids, whereas others report a worsening of symptoms; moreover, studies to date have not substantiated the efficacy of oral contraceptive steroids over placebo. It is perhaps worth noting that isolated case reports have claimed an improvement of psychotic symptoms linked to the menstrual cycle when oral contraceptive steroids have been used as a component of the treatment regimen.[14,15] Oral contraceptives do have proved effectiveness in dysmenorrhea. Therefore for women younger than age 35 with premenstrual symptoms who require contraception, and especially in those in whom dysmenorrhea is a prominent symptom, oral contraceptives may be considered for therapy. When oral contraceptives are utilized, it is usually recommended that a gestagen-dominant contraceptive be employed, although this agent worsens symptoms in some groups.

DIURETICS

Diuretics have been overutilized throughout the years for the treatment of premenstrual symptoms. Interestingly, most women who report bloating do not have documented weight gain. For women with substantiated weight gain and edema, the first step is a reduction of salt intake and refined carbohydrates. When these measures are ineffective, some have claimed that pyridoxine is efficacious. Lastly, spironolactone, an aldosterone antagonist and diuretic, has been claimed to be useful in the treatment of premenstrual symptoms,[16] but most studies have not confirmed its efficacy. However, when menstrually related edema and weight gain are persistent and a trial of diuretics appears warranted, spironolactone 25 mg qid can be utilized during the period of active symptoms.

BROMOCRIPTINE

Because of questions of possible prolactin abnormalities related to premenstrual symptoms, bromocriptine has been utilized as a treatment regimen.[17] To date, links to prolactin abnormalities remain tenuous, and benefits of bromocriptine also remain unsubstantiated. Bromocriptine is not an innucuous drug. Nausea is a frequent side effect. Patients may also experience such symptoms as headache, dizziness, or fatigue. Occasionally hypotension is noted. If there is hyperprolactinemia, further evaluation, especially to rule out a pituitary tumor, is warranted before bromocriptine treatment is indicated. Furthermore, bromocriptine may be considered for the control of breast swelling and tenderness. When utilized, the dose is 2.5 mg orally twice daily. Other medications that may be effective for the control of breast swelling and tenderness are spironolactone 25 mg orally four times daily and danazol, an antiestrogen, 200 mg orally twice daily.[5] Patients taking danazol sometimes report the development of acne, mild hirsutism, and decreased breast size. Mild hypoestrogenic manifestations are sometimes seen. There are also reports of dizziness, muscle cramps, and gastrointestinal symptoms, usually of a mild nature. Patients receiving danazol are counseled about avoiding conception during its use.

ANTIPROSTAGLANDINS

Antiprostaglandins clearly are efficacious in the treatment of dysmenorrhea. In general, however, they do not appear to have similar usefulness in the treatment of premenstrual symptoms, except perhaps for breast tenderness, abdominal bloating, ankle swelling, and edema. It is perhaps worth remembering that until a decade ago confusion around the etiology and treatment of dysmenorrhea was similar to that which now exists concerning many premenstrual symptoms. The documented pathophysiology of dysmenorrhea and the corresponding usefulness of the antiprostraglandins for its treatment lend hope and may presage development in the understanding and treatment of at least some categories of premenstrual syndromes.

Other treatment regimens and research approaches are currently being utilized in a number of medical centers. One approach is the use of a yeast-free diet combined with oral or vaginal nystatin.[13] Another is the experimental elimination of ovarian cyclicity with an agonist of gonadotropin-releasing hormone, with improvement of symptoms in a small number of cases.[18] Careful studies of these and other approaches are needed to assess their possible efficacy.

DISCUSSION

We have considered approaches to evaluation and management of the premenstrual symptoms that clinicians encounter in practice. We have undertaken this task with the knowledge that theoretical underpinnings remain questionable and that clinical research has been confounded by methodologic

problems with results for given approaches subsequently not being replicated. We recognize that future studies will provide important information
about premenstrual symptoms, including evaluation and treatment strategies
and the possible links between premenstrual syndromes and psychiatric
symptoms. Yet we are also aware that in the interim women in increasing
numbers are requesting treatment for symptoms, that sensitive clinicians are
independently linking symptoms to the menstrual cycle, and that clinicians
are employing treatment regimens—even if unverified—for these symptoms.

We stress the importantance of a careful prospective evaluation prior to
the initiation of any treatment. Significant numbers of patients require no further treatment at the end of the period of evaluation. They may learn triggering factors, methods of decreasing pressures, and self-treatment techniques. Some feel more comfortable living with their symptoms. Among
those requiring treatment, a number of patterns have become apparent.

Some women have symptoms, but with patterns apparently unrelated to
the menstrual cycle. Others, whose symptoms appear related to the menstrual cycle, warrant further assessment, and we recommend careful evaluation with emphasis on gynecologic, medical, nutritional, endocrine, neurologic, and psychiatric components. Specific findings may emerge to explain
symptoms and indicate specific treatment. We emphasize that if clinicians are
going to prescribe medications for premenstrual symptoms they must recognize that the theoretical rationale and confirmatory data remain fragmentary
and that FDA approval in most cases is lacking. We therefore advice clinicians
to be cautious and use approaches initially that appear to be pharmacologically safest, reserving other approaches for more refractory cases. We also encourage clinicians to look for side effects and provide careful follow-up to
monitor treatment efficacy.

With this in mind, we have summarized some approaches that are currently being utilized for treatment. Overall approaches incorporate exercise; a
well-balanced diet including decreased intake of refined sugars, white flour,
coffee, tea, and chocolate; decreased alcohol consumption; and cutbacks in
smoking. A number of treatment regimens include vitamins; progesterone,
either natural progesterone, synthetic derivatives, or oral contraceptive steroids; diurectics, bromocriptine, and other steroids, and antiprostaglandins.
We have provided some logical guidelines on the basis of patient symptoms,
clinical data, and research underpinnings. We hope that in future years other
conceptualizations and careful clinical studies will provide more coherent
approaches to understanding, evaluating, and treating premenstrual symptoms.

REFERENCES

1. Frank RT: Hormonal causes of premenstrual tension. Arch Neurol Psychiatry 26:
   1053, 1931
2. Rubinow DR, Roy-Byrne P: Premenstrual syndromes: overview from a methodologic perspective. Am J Psychiatry 141:163, 1984

3. Newmark NE, Penrey JK: Catamenial epilepsy. Epilepsia 21:281, 1980
4. Carr DB, et al: Physical conditioning facilitates the exercise-induced secretion of beta-endorphin and beta-lipotropin in women. N Engl J Med 305:560, 1981
5. Reid RL, Yes SS: The premenstrual syndrome. Clin Obstet Gynecol 26:710, 1983
6. Bertoli A, DePirro R, Fusco A, et al: Differences in insulin receptors between men and menstruating women and influence of sex hormones on insulin binding during the menstrual cycle. J Clin Endocrinol 50:246, 1984
7. Winston, F: Oral Contraceptives, pyridoxine, and depression. Am J Psychiatry 130:1217, 1973
8. Schaumburg H, et al: Sensory neuropathy from pyridoxine abuse. N Engl J Med 309:445, 1983
9. Berger, Allen, Schaumburg H: More on neuropathy from pyridoxine abuse (letter to the editor). N Engl J Med 311:986, 1984
10. Dalton K: The Premenstrual Syndrome and Progesterone Therapy. Heinemann, London, 1977
11. Sampson, GA: Premenstrual syndrome: a double-blind controlled trial of progesterone and placebo. Br Psychiatry 135:209, 1979
12. Smith SL: Mood and the menstrual cycle. In Sacher EJ (ed): Topics in Psychoendocrinology. p. 19. Grune & Stratton, New York, 1975
13. Schinfeld JS, Cronin L: Premenstrual syndrome. In press.
14. Felthous AR, Robinson DB, Conroy RW: Prevention of recurrent menstrual psychosis by an oral contraceptive. Am J Psychiatry 137:245, 1980
15. Glick RD, Stewart, D: A new drug treatment premenstrual exacerbation of schizophrenia. Compr Psychiatry 21:281, 1980
16. O'Brien PM, Craven D, Selby D, et al: Treatment of premenstrual syndrome by spironolactone. Br J Obstet Gynaecol 86:142, 1979
17. Andersen, AN, Larsen JF: Bromocriptine in the treatment of the premenstrual syndrome. Drugs 17:383, 1979
18. Muse K, et al: The premenstrual syndrome: effects of "medical ovariectomy." N Engl J Med 311:1345, 1984

9

Perspective from a PMS Clinic

Lorraine Dennerstein
Carol Morse
Gordon Gotts
Graham D. Burrows
James B. Brown
Margery A. Smith
Elizabeth Farrell

Premenstrual complaints affect a significant proportion of women during their reproductive years. With growing media publicity there have been increased demands from women for effective treatment. Not surprisingly in view of the current controversies surrounding all aspects of the premenstrual syndromes (PMS), some doctors are confused about therapy approaches. Specialist PMS clinics were established with the goals of providing a comprehensive approach to the health care of women presenting with premenstrual complaints. This centralization of patients and staff facilitated research and education about this disorder.

This chapter is based on our experiences with PMS clinics, all of which are attached to major teaching hospitals in Melbourne, Australia. A considerable amount of research has been conducted at these clinics over the last 5 years. Where possible, preliminary findings are included.

PMS CLINICS

The establishment of a specialist PMS clinic has many benefits. The name of the clinic allows identification of the facility to potential patients and referral sources. Centralization enables all medical and paramedical specialists involved to work together as a coordinated multidisciplinary team. The intention is to provide a total assessment of each woman, a clear, balanced picture of her descriptive and prescriptive needs. Medical screening for hypertension, diabetes, and breast and gynecologic disorders can be carried out. Hormone and other therapeutic modalities can be controlled and evaluated on both short- and long-term bases. Long-term benefits and risks can be established. This arrangement also facilitates data gathering so that the experience and expertise gained from the clinic can be shared with others. Specialist clinics have broad educational goals. Internally, education of patients corrects misinformation and provides an explanation for symptoms. The teaching hospital association of the clinic provides for teaching medical undergraduates and postgraduates as well as staff of all disciplines. An outreach educational program increases the knowledge of the community. Lectures to doctors inform them of research findings and new developments in therapies. PMS clinics fulfill many of the general goals of other specialist clinics such as menopause clinics.[1]

There are some difficulties in conducting a multidisciplinary PMS clinic.[2] Efficient team functioning depends on extensive sharing and interdependence. Each member needs a clear sense of role responsibilities and boundaries and a fundamental understanding of how they all integrate. Multidisciplinary clinics may suffer from a lack of leadership and direction if these areas are not clearly established. There may be a battle for leadership between medical specialists.

A major problem has been the inappropriateness of some referrals, for example, when a patient with chronic schizophrenia presents claiming that premenstrual tension (PMT)* is the cause of all her problems. Sometimes inappropriate referrals are patient-initiated. On other occasions doctors initiate. Both are seeking to relabel a chronic psychiatric problem. Another difficult area is the setting for a clinic. Should the clinic be attached to the gynecology division, or should it be located at community health clinics?

CLINICAL ASSESSMENT

The paucity of adequate research made it necessary for our clinic to collect as much data as possible. The following regimen was utilized.

REFERRAL

All patients were referred by their primary care doctor. Quite often assessment revealed disorders more appropriately treated outside the clinic, and liaison with the woman's doctor was needed. The problem of inappropriate referrals was partly dealt with by the utilization of a preliminary questionnaire. It was completed and returned by the patient before an appointment was made.

---

*PMT is used synonomously with PMS. It is the original terminology used by Frank in 1931 to describe these symptoms.

INITIAL EVALUATION

Patients were interviewed during the first half of the menstrual cycle. Women who suffer from PMS were often so distressed during the latter part of the cycle that it was difficult to obtain and formulate the history. Both medical and psychosocial assessments were carried out. Interviews provided demographic information on the patient, detailed complaints and their association with the menstrual cycle, past and any concurrent medical, gynecologic, and psychiatric history, social and occupational areas, and stress factors. Vulnerability to hormone-provoked symptoms was indicated by a history of post-partum depression and of mood side effects to the oral contraceptive pill. Physical, including gynecologic, examination was carried out to exclude other organic pathology.

Psychometric tests provided additional information on personality functioning. The following were utilized.

Eysenck Personality Inventory (Form B)[3]
Locus of Control Scale[4]
Self-Esteem Scale[5]
General Well-Being Scale[6]
Dyadic Adjustment Scale[7]
Attitudes to Menses and Menopause[8]

These scales have been useful in establishing a psychosocial profile of women presenting with premenstrual complaints.

PROSPECTIVE PMS EVALUATION

In order to establish a diagnosis of PMS, women were followed prospectively for two menstrual cycles. They were reinterviewed during the premenstrual phase to assess symptomatology and mental status. In order to quantify symptoms objectively, the following rating scales were administered during both the follicular (days 5 to 8) and the premenstrual (days 23 to 28) phases of the cycle: Moos Menstrual Distress Questionnaire (MDQ),[9] Beck Depression Inventory,[10] Spielberger State Anxiety Inventory,[11] and Mood Adjective Checklist.[12] Daily Symptom Ratings[13] of 10 variables were completed by the women throughout the cycle.

Daily 12- and 24-hour collections of urine throughout the menstrual cycle were performed in order to determine the role of hormonal factors in the premenstrual syndrome. Urinary total estrogens and pregnanediol were measured.[14,15] Hormonal results of the first 30 patients[16] are summarized.

PRELIMINARY RESULTS

All women aged 18 to 45 who at the initial interview reported moderate to severe mood and/or physical symptoms premenstrually were included providing they were not taking hormonal medications and had regular cycles (between 3 and 5 weeks). After being studied over two menstrual cycles women were separated into the following two groups (according to the objective and subjective assessments detailed above).

1. Premenstrual syndrome (PMS)
   a. No history of psychiatric disorder (using *DSM-III* Axis I diagnostic criteria) within the previous 12 months. Women with Axis II Personality Disorder diagnoses were not excluded.
   b. Complaints were not present continuously throughout the cycle. A symptom-free phase of at least 1 week was present.
   c. A "difference score" of more than 30 on the MDQ between follicular and premenstrual assessment.
2. Menstrual distress syndrome (MDS)
   a. Presence of a diagnosable psychiatric disorder, e.g., anxiety, affective disorder, or schizophrenia, using *DSM-III* Axis I diagnostic criteria.
   b. Presence of symptoms of at least moderate intensity throughout the cycle with exacerbation during the premenstruum.

SYMPTOMS

The 10 most frequently reported complaints were as follows.

Irritability
Depression
Painful breasts
Abdominal bloating
Weight gain
Fatigue
Aggression
Headache
Tension
Breast swelling

HORMONAL PROFILE

Results of the hormonal profile have been reported in detail elsewhere.[16] The hormonal data from 30 patients' cycles were compared with those of 84 control women. When the characteristics of a "normal" menstrual cycle were defined in terms of daily urinary total estrogen and pregnanediol excretions, 87 percent of control cycles met these hormonal criteria. Only 37 percent of patient cycles could be considered normal ($\chi^2 = 28.6$, $p < 10^{-6}$). Abnormalities in the patient groups compared with controls included lower preovulatory estrogen peak values, either high or low estrogen values during the luteal phase, short or deficient luteal phases, and a later rise in periovulatory pregnanediol. Significantly lower pregnanediol values were evident in PMS patients. Hormonal abnormalities were more marked in the PMS group than in the MDS group.

PSYCHOSOCIAL PROFILE

Psychological and demographic data of the first 80 patients to attend our clinic revealed the following (Table 9-1): The mean age of the women was 35 ± 5 years. Thirty percent were engaged in home duties primarily, and 70 percent worked full-time or part-time outside their homes. Of those who worked, 31 percent were in professional occupations and a further 49 percent in semiskilled occupations. Seventy-six percent were currently married. Median parity was 2 with a range from 0 to 5. Seventeen percent were nulliparous. In those in whom pregnancy had occurred there was a history of postpartum depression in 68 percent. In 31 percent depression had followed more than one pregnancy. Only three women had not received the oral contraceptive pill. Ninety-two percent of PMS women and 76 percent of MDS women reported side effects.

Of the 80 women, 38 suffered PMS and 42 MDS. Table 9-2 details psychometric results for the two groups. Women with MDS had significantly higher neuroticism scores. MDS patients had significantly higher scores than women with PMS on the general well-being scale for the parameter "worn out" and a tendency to report feeling more "uptight." Patients with MDS had significantly more negative attitudes about their bodies and a tendency to have more negative attitudes in general. Husbands of women with MDS were significantly less satisfied with their marriages than husbands of women with

TABLE 9-1. PMS CLINIC PATIENTS: PSYCHOSOCIAL PROFILE

Parameter	%
Total no. = 80 (PMS = 38; MDS = 42)	
Age (mean) = 35 ± 5 years	
Occupation	
Homemaker	30
Outside home (full or part time)	70
Professional	31
Semiskilled	49
Others (unskilled)	20
Marital status: married	76
Parity: median = 2 (range 0–5)	
Nulliparous	17
Postpartum depression	
Single episode	68
Recurrent	31
Oral contraceptive pills	96
Side effects	
PMS patients	92
MDS patients	76

TABLE 9-2. PSYCHOMETRIC TEST RESULTS

Parameter	PMS (*n* = 38)	MDS (*n* = 42)
Neuroticism	14.03	16.07[a]
Extraversion	13.45	12.81
L. score	1.58	1.95
Locus of control	13.16	14.21
General well-being		
Uptight	21.00	25.42
Worn out	25.00	29.83[a]
Attitudes		
Menses	8.5	7.8
Menarche	1.02	0.75
Body	3.57	3.14[a]
Genitals	3.44	3.41
Sex	5.52	5.43
Masturbation	1.42	1.29
Menopause	4.16	4.35
Dyadic adjustment		
Female		
Consensus	47.94	45.04[a]
Affection	8.11	7.54
Satisfaction	36.66	32.27
Cohesion	14.11	13.95
Total	103.52	100.50
Male		
Consensus	49.23	46.18[a]
Affection	8.15	8.53
Satisfaction	39.54	34.71
Cohesion	16.53	15.64
Total	106.86	106.63

[a]$p \leq 0.05$.

PMS. Women with MDS rated their marriages more negatively than did their partners or women with PMS. Thus women with MDS functioned less well psychologically than did PMS sufferers.

EVALUATION OF THERAPIES

Our clinics have evaluated several therapy regimens. A double-blind crossover placebo-controlled trial has been conducted for oral micronized progesterone (Utrogestan). Analysis[13] found promising results. A marked reduction in symptomatology occurred during the trial, but it was more marked during progesterone treatment. Following the trial some of the women continued hormonal medication and participated in a group treatment program that utilized rational emotive therapy* and relaxation training. Further im-

---

*Rational emotive therapy (RET) is based on assumptions that emotional difficulties are largely cognitively mediated. This therapy has been increasingly shown to be effective in the treatment of fairly intractible psychological disorders (e.g., trichotillomania).[17]

provement in symptomatology (mood, behavior, and pain); cognitive functioning and neuroticism was noted. Hormonal therapy was then withdrawn. Follow-up 3 months later showed that improvements in mood were maintained but not in symptoms of pain and water retention. This study demonstrated that the combination of cognitive behavior therapy with hormonal intervention produced a more substantial reduction in PMS symptoms than did drug treatment alone.

IMPLICATIONS FOR THE CLINICIAN

ASSESSMENT

The first major problem facing the clinician is making a diagnosis. All patients presenting with premenstrual complaints need a full assessment. It requires interviews, examination, and some quantification of symptomatology to be carried out in both follicular and premenstrual phases of the cycle. Simple assessment methods may include Daily Symptom Rating Scale (Fig. 9-1) or the Moos Menstrual Distress Questionnaire.[9]

For routine clinical management hormonal evaluation is seldom needed. Weekly determinations of ovarian steroids and gonadotropins may be helpful in the assessment of the woman with amenorrhea and cyclic complaints as well as of the perimenopausal woman. Prolactin estimations are necessary only if a pituitary lesion is suspected, e.g., the woman with galactorrhea.

Some patients appear improved by the process of assessment and state that no further therapy is required. Other women are essentially "false-positives," who rate themselves globally and remember premenstrual symptoms retrospectively but do not show premenstrual changes on daily self-reports or standardized measures. Some of these patients have primary psychiatric diagnoses. The remaining patients comprise two groups: those with a discrete premenstrual syndrome and those with symptoms of some type throughout the cycle that may be exacerbated premenstrually. In the latter group psychological factors appear to be more important, whereas in the PMS group hormonal factors are more marked (Table 9-3).

TREATMENT

A broad approach is taken when planning therapy. Our research results indicate that both psychological and hormonal factors may be important in premenstrual symptomatology. There are as yet no studies indicating if the various therapy approaches are differentially effective for PMS and MDS patients. In fact, there may be other subgroups for whom a specific treatment is preferable. This problem is a critical one for study in the future.

INFORMATION

After assessment, results are explained to the individual patient and a rationale for her symptoms offered. A general rationale explains that psychological or thinking patterns, hormonal abnormalities, and individual sensi-

Week beginning: _____

Name: _____

My last period started on: _____

Each night before retiring, please record your experience
during the day of the feelings and sensations listed below.
Write a number in the box opposite the item to indicate how
intensely this symptom or feeling was experienced.

1	2	3	4	5
Not at all	Very little	Moderate amount	A fair bit	A great deal

Date								
1. Restlessness								
2. Headache								
3. Breast discomfort								
4. Depression								
5. Active aggression								
6. Hot flushes								
7. Feelings of well-being								
8. Irritability								
9. Sexual thoughts or interest								
10. Swelling of abdomen, hands, legs								
Menstruation: No. of pads or tampons used								

Fig. 9-1. Daily symptom record.

tivity to hormone-provoked symptoms are important in the genesis and maintenance of symptoms. The role of each in the individual presentation can then be highlighted.

INTERVENTION

There is little substantive evidence of the effectiveness of the widely used medications: pyridoxine and diuretics. Most patients attending our clinics had already received these medications and reported little improvement. There was initial resistance to psychological therapy approaches. Most pa-

TABLE 9-3. PMS CLINIC PATIENTS

1. Spontaneous remission (during evaluation)
2. False-positives: state they have PMS, but premenstrual changes cannot be demonstrated (psychiatric diagnoses common)
3. PMS
4. MDS: symptoms throughout the cycle with premenstrual exacerbation

tients seem to desire hormonal intervention. Hormonal intervention with oral micronized progesterone (Utrogestan; Laboratoires Besins Iscovesco, France) 100 mg in the morning and 200 mg at night from days 17 to 27 is recommended. Open evaluation also suggests that duphaston 10 mg PO bid is well tolerated and may have beneficial effects. In contrast, the 19 nonsteroids such as norethisterone often worsen premenstrual complaints. Once an initial improvement in symptomatology has been achieved, women often became much more accessible to psychological treatment strategies. Supportive therapy and techniques aimed at increasing coping skills (and changing dysfunctional cognition) are likely to be helpful. Behavioral techniques such as relaxation and assertiveness training may also be beneficial.

SUMMARY AND CONCLUSION

Clinics for the treatment of premenstrual changes have been established to meet the demands from women for treatment of these common disorders. The conduct of a PMS clinic is described. Women taking hormonal medications and those with only mild symptoms were not included. Patients were categorized as having either PMS (no psychiatric disorder and a symptom-free period) or MDS (diagnosable psychiatric disorder and premenstrual exacerbation of continuous symptoms). Hormonal abnormalities were found in patients compared with controls and were more marked in the PMS than in the MDS group. A history of postpartum depression and side effects of oral contraceptives was common.

A trial of orally effective micronized (natural) progesterone was promising, but a combination of psychotherapy and hormonal intervention seemed preferable to drug treatment alone. The patient group was heterogeneous and included, in addition to PMS and MDS patients, women with spontaneous remission and false positives (women who complain of premenstrual symptoms in whom no such changes can be demonstrated). Both psychological and hormonal factors seem important in the etiology and treatment of PMS. The elucidation of subgroups for whom specific treatment is effective is an important goal.

REFERENCES

1. Utian WH: Menopause clinics; purpose, function and international comparisons. p. 147. In van Keep PA, Utian WH, Vermenler A (eds): The Controversial Climacteric. MTP Press, Lancaster, 1982

2. Morse C, Dennerstein L, Farrell E: Menstrual–menopause problems: a team approach patient management. In press, 1984
3. Eysenck HJ, Eysenck SBG: Manual of the Eysenck Personality Inventory. Hodder & Stoughton, Kent, 1964
4. James WH: Internal vs external control of reinforcement as a basic variable in learning theory. Doctoral dissertation, Ohio State University, 1957
5. Rosenberg M: Society and the Adolescent Self-Image. Princeton University Press, Princeton, 1965
6. Cox T, Thirlaway M, Gotts G, Cox S: The nature and assessment of general well-being. J Psychosom Res. In press, 1984
7. Spanier GB: New scales for assessing the quality of marriage and similar dyads. J Marriage Family Feb:15, 1976
8. Spencer-Gardner C, Dennerstein L, Burrows GD: Premenstrual tension and the female role. J Psychosom Obstet Gynaecol 2:27, 1983
9. Moos RH: The development of a menstrual distress questionnaire. Psychosom Med 30:853, 1968
10. Beck AT, Ward CH, Mendelson M, et al: An inventory for measuring depression. Arch Gen Psychiatry 4:561, 1961
11. Spielberger CD, Gorusch RL, Lushere RE: Manual for the State-Trait Anxiety. Consulting Psychologists Press, Palo Alto, 1970
12. Mackey C, Cox T, Burrows G, Lazzerini T: An inventory for the measurement of self-reported stress and arousal. Br J Soc Clin Psychol 17:283
13. Dennerstein L, Spencer-Gardner C, Gotts G, et al: Progesterone and the premenstrual syndrome: a double-blind cross-over trial. Br Med J. In press, 1985
14. Brown JB, Macleod SC, Macnaughton C, et al: A rapid method for estimating oestrogen in wine taking using a semi-automatic extractor. J Endocrinol 42:5, 1968
15. Barrett SA, Brown, JB: An evaluation of the method of Cox for the rigid analysis of pregnanediol in wine by gas-liquid chromatography. J Endocrinol 47:471, 1970
16. Dennerstein L, Spencer-Gardner C, Brown JB, et al: Premenstrual tension—hormonal profiles. J Psychosom Obstet Gynaecol 3:37, 1984
17. Bernard ME, Kratochwill TR, Keefauver LW: The effects of rational-emotive therapy and self-instructional training on chronic hair-pulling. Cognitive Ther Res 7:273, 1983
18. Morse C, Bernard M, Dennerstein L: The effects of rational emotive therapy and relaxation training on premenstrual symptomatology—a preliminary study. In press, 1984
19. Dennerstein L, Burrows G: Psychological effects of progestins in the menopausal years. In press, 1984

10

Progesterone: Biologic Effects and Evaluation of Therapy for PMS

Wayne S. Maxson

Although the premenstrual syndromes continue to confound systematic scientific inquiry, multiple therapies have been championed as palliative or curative. Various treatment modalities have received anecdotal acclaim, but few have proved more effective than placebo in controlled, prospective treatment trials.

Progesterone therapy holds a unique position in the annals of the premenstrual syndromes, due primarily to the singular efforts of Dalton.[1] This chapter reviews the pharmacology and physiology of progesterone, theories relating to the possible efficacy of progesterone in the treatment of premenstrual syndrome (PMS), and a summary of the current literature regarding clinical trials of progesterone for treatment of premenstrual disorders.

HISTORY OF PROGESTERONE THERAPY FOR PMS

Progesterone was first used to treat PMS in 1934, the same year that this hormone was isolated.[2] From the 1930s to the 1970s, intermittent, uncontrolled reports advocated progesterone therapy by suppository, pessary, or injection.[3-8]

In 1977 and 1984 Dalton gave progesterone therapy new impetus in two editions of *The Premenstrual Syndrome and Progesterone Therapy*.[1] Her enthusiasm and the personal experience of a number of PMS sufferers led to the formation in 1979 in Madison, Wisconsin, of PMS Action, Inc., the first nonprofit consumer organization concerned with PMS in the United States (now located in Irvine, CA).[9] In addition to the dissemination of information about PMS and the expansion of consumer support for PMS study, PMS Action, Inc. perpetuated interest in progesterone as an effective therapy for PMS sufferers who did not benefit from other treatment modalities.

In 1984 Lyon and Lyon conducted a survey of treatment practices for PMS.[10] In this study the authors mailed questionnaires to 1,597 physicians in the United States and Canada, obtaining their names from PMS Action, Inc. Of the 503 responses, 502 were deemed usable for analysis. Progesterone was the most widely recommended treatment, advocated by 69.9 percent of respondents.[10]

Despite widespread use of progesterone for premenstrual syndromes, most clinicians and researchers remain puzzled about the true role of this steroid for the treatment of these cryptic conditions. An understanding of the physiology and pharmacology of progesterone and a critical review of the literature on its use are important foundations for physicians and patients interested in the diagnosis and treatment of these cyclic premenstrual disorders.

THE PROGESTERONE HYPOTHESIS

PROGESTERONE DEFICIENCY

In the 1981 *A Guide to Progesterone Therapy for PMS*, Dalton stated that "PMS is a progesterone deficiency disease, responding to progesterone replacement therapy."[9] This progesterone imbalance has been hypothesized to result from: (1) a relative deficiency in progesterone production by the corpus luteum; (2) an alteration in the normal estrogen/progesterone ratio; (3) premature progesterone withdrawal; and (4) an endogenous allergy to progesterone (Table 10-1).

A systematic evaluation of serum progesterone concentrations during the luteal phase in PMS sufferers has been scientifically impractical, because of the remarkable fluctuation in progesterone levels consequent to the pulsatile secretion of this steroid hormone. Filicori and colleagues demonstrated widely varying progesterone levels ranging from 5 to 35 ng/ml over a 12-hour period during the midluteal phase in normal volunteers.[11] Single, or even several, progesterone measurements may therefore be poorly reflective of the total progesterone output or availability during the luteal phase. Serum progesterone levels also correlate poorly with active tissue concentrations of this hormone and with the cellular concentrations of progesterone receptors. Not surprisingly, of 10 controlled investigations of blood progesterone levels in PMS patients from 1974 to 1981, six reported lower progesterone levels during

TABLE 10-1.   PROGESTERONE HYPOTHESES FOR PMS

Progesterone deficiency
    Abnormal corpus luteum
    Decreased receptors
    Increased protein binding

Progesterone hypersensitivity

Estrogen abnormality
    Abnormal corpus luteum

the midluteal phase,[12-17] one showed elevated progesterone concentrations,[18] and three showed no abnormality in progesterone secretion.[19-21]

PROGESTERONE ALLERGY

Gerber in 1921[22] and Urbach in 1939[23] demonstrated that premenstrual urticaria could be caused by hypersensitivity to a substance in the blood. Experimentally, the reinjection of serum from affected individuals reproduced the urticaria, and desensitization by repeated small injections of this serum resulted in a cure.[24] Zondek and Bromberg suggested that PMS could be caused by actual sensitivity to progesterone.[25,26]

A variety of other disorders have been attributed to an endogenous allergy to progesterone, including premenstrual asthma, dermatitis, and eczema.[27-29] Immunofluorescence techniques have demonstrated antibodies to progesterone in affected individuals.[29]

ESTROGEN ABNORMALITY

Because estrogen often appears to oppose the actions of progesterone, the estrogen hypothesis has been popular since Frank in 1931 first ascribed PMS to abnormal estrogen secretion.[30] Alterations in estrogen production, metabolism, or binding can reduce the circulating levels of free, biologically active estrogen and alter the estrogen/progesterone ratio and the tissue concentration of progesterone receptors during the luteal phase.

Early studies estimated the estrogen effect by karyopyknotic indices in vaginal smears or by endometrial biopsies.[31,32] Measurement of estradiol levels during the luteal phase in PMS sufferers, however, has produced variable results. Whereas four studies reported elevated estrogen concentrations during the late luteal phase,[16,17,32,33] four other studies have shown normal estrogen concentrations during the mid and late luteal phases.[13,19-21]

An alteration in binding protein can influence the amount of free, and therefore active, estrogen and progesterone in the circulation. Dalton in 1981 reported that PMS patients have lower sex hormone binding globulin capacity during the premenstruum than controls.[34] However, other investigators have been unable to detect a change in hormone binding globulin during the luteal phase.[35-37]

SITE OF PROGESTERONE PRODUCTION IN WOMEN

The adrenal gland produces progesterone from cholesterol and pregnenolone as an intermediate in the biosynthesis of corticosteroids, in quantities of 0.75 mg per day.[38,39] During the proliferative phase of the menstrual cycle, most of the circulating progesterone is adrenal in origin.[40] Follicular phase concentrations of progesterone in serum generally range between 0.1 and 1.0 ng/ml.

During the luteal phase, progesterone production by the ovarian corpus luteum is dramatic and may reach 50 mg per day.[40] During the midluteal phase, at the time of expected implantation of the conceptus, serum progesterone concentrations average 5 to 25 ng/ml.

During pregnancy the placenta contributes an additional 25 to 40 mg of progesterone per day. Progesterone concentrations during gestation progressively increase to a mean of 175 ng/ml at term.[42]

PROGESTERONE METABOLISM

First crystallized in 1934 by a number of researchers and subsequently named in 1935,[38] progesterone is pregn-4-ene-3,20-dione in systematic nomenclature. Secreted by the adrenal gland, corpus luteum, and placental trophoblast, an identical steroid can also be synthesized from certain plants, especially the Mexican yam. Progesterone today is commercially available from these inexpensive plant sources.

Progesterone itself is the most potent progestogen, but enzymatic degradation of progesterone produces a plethora of metabolites with varying progestational actions and other biologic effects.[41]

In the circulation the half-life of progesterone has been measured as 19 minutes.[43] Like other steroids, progesterone is rapidly degraded in the peripheral circulation as well as in various tissues.

The specific metabolism of progesterone depends on the site of metabolic breakdown. For example, the corpus luteum produces substantial amounts of 17-hydroxyprogesterone during the luteal phase. 17-Hydroxyprogesterone concentrations reach 2.5 ng/ml during the midluteal phase.[42] During pregnancy, however, only a modest increase in 17-hydroxyprogesterone levels occurs despite prodigious ovarian and placental production of progesterone, indicating a low activity of 17α-hydroxylase in placental trophoblast.[42]

The most constant metabolite of progesterone is 20α-hydroxyprogesterone (20α-hydroxypregen-4-ene-3-one). This form of progesterone is largely an inactive metabolite.

In the brain certain sites associated with the behavioral effects of progesterone (e.g., the midbrain) contain increased concentrations of 5α-reductase enzymes, which convert progesterone to 5α-dihydroprogesterone (5α-pregnane-3,20-dione).[44]

BIOLOGIC EFFECTS OF PROGESTERONE

Progesterone is a potent steroid with diverse effects on many cells and organ systems (Table 10-2). Progesterone, like other steroids, rapidly diffuses across the plasma membranes of the cells. Evidence indicates that progesterone is bound to nuclear receptors and modulates cellular protein synthesis as a result of the receptor–nucleus interaction.

Progesterone also exhibits more rapid and direct effects on cell membranes independent of protein synthesis. One example is the effect on the

TABLE 10-2. BIOLOGIC EFFECTS OF PROGESTERONE

System	Effect
Uterus	
Myometrium	Growth
	Inhibition of contractions
Endometrium	Secretory changes
	Decidualization of stroma
	Uteroglobin synthesis
Breast	Growth
	Acinar development
	Inhibition of lactalbumin
Kidney	Inhibition of aldosterone receptor binding
	Increased sodium excretion by tubules
Smooth muscle	Relaxation
Cell membranes	Inhibition of prostaglandin synthesis by stabilization of lysosomes
	Stimulus of prostaglandin synthetase
	Increase in intracellular calcium in frog oocyte
Brain	Sedation or anesthesia
	Increased seizure threshold
	Competition for GABA-barbiturate receptor
	Increased MAO activity
	Altered serotonin turnover
	Increased endogenous opiates
	Thermogenic shift
	Modulation of GnRH
Adenohypophysis	Modulation of gonadotropin and prolactin secretion

frog oocyte, where progesterone causes a rapid and transient increase in intracellular calcium associated with the reinitiation of meiosis.[45] Progesterone has also been found to exert an extremely rapid effect (in milliseconds) on nerve cell membrane conductivity in the brain.

UTERUS

In conjunction with estradiol, progesterone stimulates the growth of the uterus and induces a number of specific changes in the endometrium and myometrium. In an endometrium primed with estrogen, progesterone causes differentiation of the uterine lining from a proliferative to a secretory pattern. Within the secretory endometrium, progesterone stimulates an increase in intracellular glycogen, part of the process of decidualization required for implantation of the conceptus.

Progesterone induces secretion of the protein uteroglobin into the lumen of the uterus.[46] Progesterone has also been found to inhibit myometrial contractions.[38] These actions of progesterone are direct, as confirmed by multiple experiments in vitro.[38]

KIDNEY

Progesterone has been found to inhibit the binding of aldosterone to renal receptors.[47] In nonpregnant women progesterone can increase sodium excretion by direct competitive inhibition of aldosterone at the renal tubule.[48]

PROSTAGLANDINS

Progesterone priming is necessary for the stimulation of uterine prostaglandin production by estrogen.[49] However, the combination of estrogen and progesterone inhibits prostaglandin production.[49]

Progesterone may inhibit both the production of prostaglandins and their end-organ effect in several ways. Progesterone has been described to directly inhibit the binding of prostaglandin $F_{2\alpha}$ to the cell membrane of the corpus luteum.[50]

In addition, progesterone seems to stabilize the lysosomes that contain phospholipase A_2, enzymes that free arachidonic acid and initiate the cascade of prostaglandin synthesis from this precursor. At least in the placental amnion, progesterone inhibits the release of arachidonic acid through this mechanism.[51]

MUSCLE

Progesterone also has an inhibitory effect on smooth muscle.[52] In addition to relaxation of uterine myometrium,[52] progesterone has been credited for the dilatation of the ureters[53] and possibly for peripheral venous dilatation[38] during pregnancy.

BREASTS

Progesterone is a key hormone in the generation of glandular tissue in the breast. The primary effect of progesterone is on acinar growth. In conjunction with estrogen and other hormones and factors, progesterone stimulates breast growth and prepares for lactation during pregnancy. Prior to delivery, progesterone also decreases breast production of lactalbumin, thereby contributing to the inhibition of lactation prior to delivery.[54]

BRAIN

Specific receptors for progesterone are present in many areas of the brain. In rats the highest progesterone concentrations are in the cerebral cortex and the hypothalamus.[55] Progesterone is selectively taken up in the arcuate suprachiasmatic and ventromedial nuclei of the hypothalamus.[56]

The hypothalamus, like the endometrium, has a high density of progesterone receptors.[57] It is important to note that in neither organ have correlations between plasma and tissue concentrations of progesterone been shown.[58,59]

In the monkey the brain metabolically clears as much as 6 percent of circulating progesterone.[44] When progesterone concentrations are measured in the brain and the carotid artery, levels in the brain are two to five times higher than in the artery, confirming hormonal concentration within the central nervous system.[55]

Progesterone may be used as an anesthetic agent in animals and humans.[60] An intravenous dose of progesterone, 250 to 500 mg, induces sleep in normal volunteers.[60]

Certain metabolites of progesterone are more potent anesthetics than progesterone itself.[61] Majewska and colleagues[62] demonstrated that 3α-hydroxy-5α-dihydroprogesterone is a potent modulator of the γ-aminobutyric acid (GABA) receptor complex of the brain. This progesterone metabolite actively competes with barbiturates for this receptor.

Gyermek and colleagues[63] compared the potency of various progesterone metabolites with pentobarbitone sodium in a rat model. In these studies the minimum effective dose of progesterone or its metabolites that induced sleep spindles on the electroencephalogram (EEG) in cats was determined. Pregnanolone was found to be 12 times more potent than pentobarbitone, and pregnanediol and pregnanedione were three times as potent as this barbiturate. As noted in Table 10-3, pregnanolone exerted its effect immediately, whereas progesterone's sleep-inducing effect was delayed 5 to 15 minutes, suggesting a requirement for metabolism of progesterone prior to its anesthetic effect.[63]

Progesterone also has been shown to decrease interictal spikes on the EEG of cats with a penicillin-induced epileptic focus.[64] Certain metabolites of progesterone dramatically reduce the epileptic EEG spikes in the cat model, particularly 5α-pregnane-3,20-dione and 3α-hydroxy-5α-pregnane-20-one, which are 25 and 200 times as potent as progesterone, respectively.[64] In women with focal epilepsy, seizure frequency is reduced during the luteal phase.[64] These metabolites may also play a role in the central nervous system at physiologic levels, as the enzymes necessary for the production of these metabolites are identifiable in studies of rat brain.[65]

Progesterone also has an effect on catecholamines in the brain. In the rat hypothalamus progesterone increases monoamine oxidase activity and alters serotonin turnover.[66,67]

Progesterone may effect endogenous opiate activity as well. Oral contra-

TABLE 10-3.   RELATIVE ANESTHETIC POTENCY OF
PROGESTERONE METABOLITES

Agent	Activity	Time to Effect (min)
Pentobarbitone sodium	1	Immediate
Progesterone	0–3	5–15
Pregnanediol	3	2
Pregnanedione	3	2
Pregnanolone	12	Immediate

ceptives are associated with a consistent increase in the endogenous opioid peptides.[68] In addition, progestins alone have been demonstrated to increase endogenous opiate activity.[69]

LIVER

Progesterone is also metabolized and secreted in the liver. When radioactive progesterone is administered, 30 percent can be recovered in the bile.[70] Most of this progesterone is usually sulfated or glucuronidated.

Unlike synthetic progestins, natural progesterone appears to have no effect on sex hormone binding globulin, pregnancy-zone protein, or subfractions of high density lipoprotein.[71]

CONTROLLED CLINICAL TRIALS OF PROGESTERONE FOR PMS

Progesterone has been administered for treatment of PMS by various routes (including intramuscular, rectal, vaginal, subcutaneous, sublingual, nasal, and oral) and in various forms (suppository, suspension, pessary, or gelatin capsule) (Table 10-4). Clinical trials have been plagued by inherent methodologic flaws, high placebo response rates, and the vagaries of subjective measures of treatment success.

INTRAMUSCULAR ADMINISTRATION

Smith et al.[72] in 1975 evaluated the effectiveness of intramuscular progesterone (50 mg given on alternate days from cycle day 19 until menses) in a placebo-controlled trial of 14 women with premenstrual depression (Table 10-5). Ratings of depression on mood scales failed to reveal a significant beneficial effect of progesterone.

The intramuscular route has not been clinically used by most women because of the inconvenience and discomfort of this method of administration.

TABLE 10-4. ROUTES OF PROGESTERONE ADMINISTRATION

Vehicle	Route
Pessary	Vaginal
Suppository	Vaginal
	Rectal
Suspension	Rectal
	Nasal
	Sublingual
	Transcutaneous
	Oral
	Intramuscular
	Subcutaneous
Pellet	Subcutaneous

TABLE 10-5. PLACEBO-CONTROLLED TRIALS OF PROGESTERONE FOR
TREATMENT OF PMS

Authors	Subjects	Dose (mg)	Route	Duration	Results
Smith (1975)[72]	14 Women with premenstrual depression	50	IM qod	Day 19 to menses	No difference from placebo on mood scales
Sampson (1979)[74]	32 Women with PMS (Moos MDQ)	200	Rectal or vaginal bid	13 Days premenstrual × 1 cycle; other cycle placebo	No difference between progesterone and placebo at either dose
	24 Women with PMS	400	Rectal or vaginal bid	13 Days premenstrual × 1 cycle; other cycle placebo	
Keith (1985)[77]	22 Women with PMS (Keith scale)	100–200	Rectal or vaginal tid	13 Days premenstrual × 3 cycles in 11 women; 11 women received placebo × 3 cycles	No difference in psychological or somatic symptoms
Van der Meer (1983)[78]	13 Women with PMS	200	Rectal bid	Luteal phase of 2 cycles progesterone; 2 cycles placebo	No difference in psychological or somatic symptoms
Maddocks (1986)[79]	20 women with PMS	200	Vaginal bid	Luteal phase of 3 cycles progesterone; 3 cycles placebo	No difference in affective or somatic symptoms
Dennerstein (1985)[80]	23 Women with PMS	30	Oral micronized	100 mg qAM and 200 mg qPM luteal phase for 2 cycles; placebo for 2 cycles	Significant improvement over placebo in anxiety, depression, stress, swelling, fluid retention, and hot flushes

RECTOVAGINAL ADMINISTRATION

Despite enthusiastic endorsement and almost 30 years' use of rectovaginal progesterone therapy for PMS by Dalton, the studies resulting from her extensive experience are uncontrolled and inadequately documented.[73]

Sampson[74] in 1979 reported the first placebo-controlled, double-blind trial of rectovaginal progesterone for PMS (Table 10-5). In this study, 32 women with PMS, diagnosed by the Moos Menstrual Distress Questionnaire (MDQ),[75] were treated with progesterone 200 mg twice a day vaginally or rectally by suppository or pessary. After a drug-free observation cycle, progesterone was given for an average of 13 days premenstrually for one cycle, and placebo was administered for another cycle in crossover design. For the next 2 months progesterone was administered in a double-blind, controlled fashion at a dose of 400 mg twice a day for 1 month and placebo for the other month. On analysis, no significant difference between progesterone and placebo was observed by either patient retrospective self-assessment or the

MDQ daily prospective rating. Side effects of therapy in this study included rectal or vaginal discomfort, *Candida* infection, nausea, and abdominal pain on pessary insertion. The side effects were equally distributed between progesterone and placebo cycles.

The MDQ, however, has certain limitations as an analytic tool. Although this retrospective questionnaire was the only available menstrually related symptom rating scale until recently, most of its 47 items focus on somatic changes rather than mood and behavioral changes. Furthermore, it lacks specific inclusion and exclusion criteria. Finally, it was standardized on a normative sample of women, half of whom were taking oral contraceptives and almost 10 percent of whom were pregnant.[75] Only recently has a better scale been developed to assess menstrual cycle symptoms.[76]

In 1985 Keith[77] presented further data on 22 women in a placebo-controlled, double-blind study of progesterone suppository treatment of PMS (Table 10-5). Eleven women received 3 months of progesterone in a polyethylene glycol base 100 or 200 mg tid for an average of 13.2 days during the luteal phase, and 11 women received placebo three times a day for 3 months. Despite increased serum progesterone levels during progesterone treatment cycles, no significant difference in the severity of premenstrual symptoms was observed between progesterone-treated and placebo-treated patients.

Van der Meer and associates[78] in 1983 published results of a double-blind, crossover, placebo-controlled trial of rectal progesterone 200 mg in a fatty base (Table 10-5). Progesterone was given twice a day for treatment of PMS in 20 patients.[78] Daily symptoms were recorded, and an average of the scores for the 7 days prior to menses was used for statistical analysis. In this study, in a random sequence, progesterone was used for two successive cycles and placebo for two successive cycles. In the 13 patients completing the trial, no difference in psychological or somatic symptoms was detected.

In 1986 Maddocks and co-workers,[79] utilizing rigorous criteria for the selection of women with severe PMS, compared progesterone 200 mg in a polyethylene glycol base twice a day vaginally with placebo in a double-blind crossover study. Following a single control month without therapy, progesterone or placebo was given during the luteal phase for 3 consecutive months. The opposite medicine was then given for 3 consecutive months, and a final drug-free observation month ended the study. Of 48 women initially entering the study, 20 completed the protocol with data available for analysis. No significant difference between progesterone and placebo in somatic or affective symptoms was seen on the Beck Depression Inventory, MDQ, Spielberger STAI-state test, and the Buss Durkhee irritability score.

ORAL ROUTE

In 1985, using an oral preparation of micronized progesterone combined with oil in a soft gelatin capsule, Dennerstein and associates[80] performed a double-blind, placebo-controlled, crossover trial of PMS therapy. Twenty-three women with PMS, diagnosed on the basis of daily symptom recording, were treated with oral progesterone 100 mg in the morning and 200 mg at night for 10 days during the luteal phase of two consecutive cycles. In a randomized fashion, placebo was given for another two consecutive cycles.

When the mean total scores on the MDQ for all patients were plotted for progesterone therapy and compared to placebo therapy, a statistically significant benefit of progesterone for both somatic and psychological symptoms was seen. Statistically significant improvement was noted in anxiety, depression, stress, swelling, fluid retention, and hot flushes. No differential effect was seen in libido and restlessness premenstrually.*

In this study the only serious side effect was the occurrence of severe premenstrual migraine headaches on progesterone therapy. Lane and colleagues,[81] however[81] in a group of menopausal women on estrogen therapy (conjugated estrogen 1.25 mg daily) noted a PMS-like syndrome induced in 13 percent and 17 percent of patients receiving 100 mg or 300 mg of oral progesterone, respectively.

In the extensive clinical experience of Dr. J. Hargrove and myself, drowsiness and dizziness may accompany up to one-third of cycles treated with oral micronized progesterone.

PROGESTERONE DESENSITIZATION

Heckel reported an 80 percent overall relief of premenstrual symptomatology in 288 patients using small doses of pregnanediol.[82] Unfortunately, the controls were inadequate, and the diagnosis of PMS was not rigorously established in these subjects.

Maybray and colleagues[83] reported a 90 percent improvement in premenstrual symptoms by administering minute doses of aqueous progesterone suspension subcutaneously in 132 women. Improvement was evaluated by self-report, and interpretation of this study is hampered by poor pretreatment screening (sample selection) and inadequate controls.

TERATOGENICITY

Exogenous progestational agents may be teratogenic during early pregnancy (Table 10-6),[84-87] and the Food and Drug Administration (FDA) has not approved either synthetic or natural progestins for use during gestation. Two syndromes have been reported possibly related to the use of progestins during early pregnancy.

Lorber and associates[84] in 1979 reported a syndrome they called the "embryo-fetal exogenous sex steroid exposure syndrome" (EFESSES). In 9 of 16 cases evaluated, children exhibited similar dysmorphic features, including moderate growth retardation, mild to severe mental retardation, facial elongation with frontal bossing, primary telecanthus, a broad, flat nose, pouting lower lip, square chin, umbilical eversion, and external genital abnormalities in male patients. Of note, only one of these nine women received natural pro-

---

*Limitations of this study include a 1-month baseline, the use of the MDQ, the use of multiple *t*-tests, and the marked placebo response. With so many variables some *t*-tests would be expected to show significance by chance. A multiple regression analysis would be preferred to determine which variables account for the differences observed.

TABLE 10-6. POTENTIAL TERATOGENICITY OF PROGESTINS

Limb reduction defects

Genital ambiguity

Embryo-fetal exogenous sex steroid exposure syndrome (EFESSES)

Teratogen-associated cardiac syndrome (TACS)

gesterone therapy—a woman who was also taking conjugated estrogens from 4 to 12 weeks since the last menses.

Nora and associates[85] reviewed the literature on the occurrence of major anomalies in the offspring of women receiving female sex hormones. The teratogen-associated cardiac syndrome (TACS), previously called the VACTERL syndrome, appears to be increased in such offspring. These authors estimate that the risk of a major anomaly for a hormone-exposed pregnancy is 5 percent, compared to a 2 to 3 percent risk overall of major anomalies recognized at birth in the United States.

Based on available data, it is unlikely that the use of natural progesterone during early pregnancy would cause an increase in congenital anomalies, particularly in light of the marked elevations of this steroid during normal pregnancy. Nevertheless, the lack of FDA approval for this use of natural progesterone renders the administration of progesterone to women of reproductive age medically ill-advised unless an effective method of contraception is employed.

CRITICAL EVALUATION OF PROGESTERONE THERAPY FOR PMS

Progesterone, in physiologic or pharmacologic doses, is capable of producing a number of changes potentially beneficial to PMS sufferers. Theoretical advantages of progesterone include aldosterone antagonism (potentially relieving edema and bloating), smooth muscle relaxation, decreased prostaglandin production (potentially diminishing dysmenorrhea, nausea, vomiting, and diarrhea), and sedation.

The effects of the many progesterone metabolites are largely unknown, and any benefit that progesterone may render may be due more to its metabolites than to the parent steroid itself. With a broad range of somatic and psychological effects, progesterone therapy for PMS does not need to be rationalized only on the basis of the replacement of a specific steroid deficit. Pharmacologic doses of progesterone may exhibit beneficial, nonphysiologic effects.

Despite the widespread clinical use of progesterone therapy for PMS and staunch advocates of the rectovaginal route of administration, no well-designed study of rectovaginal progesterone for PMS has shown a significant difference from placebo.

Critics of these studies claim that the dosages of progesterone used are inadequate. However, studies of the absorption of rectovaginal progesterone have revealed markedly variable serum concentrations of progesterone, with only minimal increments noted after large increases in rectovaginal doses over 400 mg. The possibility that specific progesterone metabolites account for the variable efficacy of this therapeutic regimen is currently under investigation.

The beneficial effects of oral progesterone, as reported by Dennerstein, are subject to similar criticism. On the one hand, the apparent beneficial effect may represent the way in which the data were grouped and analyzed.* On the other hand, the high progesterone concentrations seen with oral progesterone therapy may indeed have provided a clinical benefit not observed with rectovaginal preparations. Alternatively, the metabolism of oral progesterone may be different from that given rectovaginally, as suggested by the increased incidence of central nervous system side effects noted anecdotally.

As of 1987, the efficacy of progesterone therapy for PMS remains to be proved. Despite this fact, progesterone remains in widespread clinical use. When taken rectovaginally, progesterone has been thought to be an expensive but safe preparation. Dalton[1] has reported no severe complications of rectal or vaginal progesterone therapy, and none have been reported in the literature to date. Long-term studies of vaginal and cervical epithelial changes and uterine and breast abnormalities are needed.

Early experience with the oral route of progesterone administration suggests that this method may not provide the margin of safety inherent in rectal and vaginal use. Hargrove and Maxson[88] have reported the case of a woman in whom deep sleep was induced by a single dose of 400 mg of oral micronized progesterone. The potential for overdose, not previously observed with rectal or vaginal progesterone administration, mandates caution in prescribing the oral route of administration. A complicating factor is the high incidence of major depression, including suicide potential, in young women. Furthermore, significant overlap between major affective disorder and the premenstrual syndromes has been demonstrated. Finally, long-term side effects with oral progesterone are as yet unknown.

Despite the likelihood that natural progesterone by any route is not teratogenic, the medicolegal risk remains. The use of high-dose progesterone for the treatment of PMS is unproved and in women exposed to pregnancy remains ill-advised. Barrier or other nonhormonal contraception is recommended for women of reproductive age receiving this therapy for PMS.

REFERENCES

1. Dalton K: The Premenstrual Syndrome and Progesterone Therapy. 2nd Ed. Yearbook, Chicago, 1984
2. Wintersteiner O, Allen WM: Crystalline progestin. J Biol Chem 107:321, 1934
3. Israel SL: Premenstrual tension. JAMA 110:1721, 1938
4. Gray LA: The use of progesterone in nervous tension states. South Med J 34:1004, 1941

---

*This study has certain problems, i.e., an evaluation period of only 1 month; use of the MDQ, which has limitations; statistical analysis using multiple *t*-tests rather than multiple regression analysis; and significant placebo response.

5. Greene R, Dalton K: The premenstrual syndrome. Br Med J 2:1007, 1953
6. Mukherjee C: Premenstrual tension: a critical study of the syndrome. J Indian Med Assoc 24:81, 1954
7. Waxman D: Progesterone and premenstrual tension syndrome. Br Med J 4:188, 1968
8. Norris RV: Progesterone for premenstrual tension. J Reprod Med 28:509, 1983
9. Dalton K: A Guide to Progesterone Therapy for Premenstrual Syndrome. PMS Action, Irvine, CA, 1981
10. Lyon KE, Lyon MA: The premenstrual syndrome: a survey of current treatment practices. J Reprod Med 29:705, 1984
11. Filicori M, Butler JP, Crowley WF: Neuroendocrine regulation of the corpus luteum in the human: evidence of pulsatile progesterone secretion. J Clin Invest 73:1638, 1984
12. Backstrom T, Carstensen H: Estrogen and progesterone in plasma relation to premenstrual tension. J Steroid Biochem 5:257, 1974
13. Smith SL: Mood in the menstrual cycle. In Sacher EH (ed): Topics in Psychoendocrinology. Grune & Stratton, Orlando, FL, 1975
14. Backstrom T, Carstensen H, Sodergard R: Concentration of estradiol, testosterone and progesterone in cerebrospinal fluid, compared to plasma unbound and total concentrations. J Steroid Biochem 7:469, 1976
15. Munday M: Hormone levels in severe premenstrual tension. Curr Med Res Opin, suppl. 4, 4:16, 1977
16. Abraham GE, Elsner CW, Lucas LA: Hormonal and behavioral changes during the menstrual cycle. Senologia 3:33, 1978
17. Munday MR, Brush MG, Taylor RW: Correlations between progesterone, oestradiol and aldosterone levels in the premenstrual syndrome. Clin Endocrinol (Oxf) 14:1, 1981
18. O'Brien PMS, Selby C, Symonds EM: Progesterone, fluid and electrolytes in premenstrual syndrome. Br Med J 1:1161, 1980
19. Andersch B, Abrahamsson L, Wendestam C: Hormone profile in premenstrual tension: effects of bromocriptine and diuretics. Clin Endocrinol (Oxf) 11:657, 1979
20. Andersen AN, Larsen JF, Steenstrup OR: Effect of bromocriptine on the premenstrual syndrome: a double-blind clinical trial. Br J Obstet Gynaecol 84:370, 1977
21. Taylor JW: Plasma progesterone, oestradiol 17 beta and premenstrual symptoms. Acta Psychiatr Scand 60:76, 1979
22. Gerber J: Einiges zur Pathologic der Urticaria menstruals. Dermatol Z 32:143, 1921
23. Urbach E: Menstruation allergy. N Int Clin 2:160, 1939
24. Gerber J: Desensitization in the treatment of menstrual intoxication and other allergic symptoms. Br J Dermatol 51:265, 1939
25. Zondek B, Bromberg YM: Endocrine allergy. J Allergy Clin Immunol 16:1, 1945
26. Zondek B, Bromberg YM: Clinical reactions of allergy to endogenous hormones and their treatment. Br J Obstet Gynaecol 54:1, 1947
27. Shelley WB, Preucel RW, Spoont SS: Autoimmune progesterone dermatitis—cure by oophorectomy. JAMA 190:147, 1964
28. Jones WN, Gordon VH: Autoimmune progesterone eczema—an endogenous progesterone hypersensitivity. Arch Dermatol 99:57, 1969
29. Farah FS, Shbaklu A: Autoimmune progesterone urticaria. J Allergy Clin Immunol 48:257, 1971
30. Frank RT: Hormonal causes of premenstrual tension. Arch Neurol Psychiatry 26:1053, 1931

31. Morton JH: Premenstrual tension. Am J Obstet Gynecol 60:343, 1950
32. Widholm OM, Tenhunen T, Hortling H: Gynecological findings in adolescence: a study of 514 patients. Acta Obstet Gynecol Scand 46:1, 1967
33. Backstrom T, Wide L, Sodergard R, et al: FSH, LH, TeBG-capacity, estrogen and progesterone in women with premenstrual tension during the luteal phase. J Steroid Biochem 7:473, 1976
34. Dalton M: Sex hormone-binding globulin levels in women with severe premenstrual syndrome. Postgrad Med J 57:560, 1981
35. Backstrom T: Epileptic seizures in women in relation to variations of plasma estrogen and progesterone during the menstrual cycle. Acta Neurol Scand 54:321, 1976
36. Backstrom T: Premenstrual tension syndrome. In Bardin CW, Milgrom E, Mauvais-Jarvis P (eds): Progesterone and Progestins. p. 203. Raven Press, New York, 1981
37. Keith GE, Spellacy WH: The use of the Keith assessment of menstrual symptomatology. Paper presented at the meeting of the International Symposium on Premenstrual Tension and Dysmenorrhea, Kiawah Island, SC, 1983
38. Little AB, Billiar RB: Progestagens. p. 92. In Fuchs F, Klopper A (eds): Endocrinology of Pregnancy. Harper & Row, Cambridge, 1983
39. Strott CA, Yoshimi T, Lipsett MB: Plasma progesterone and 17-hydroxprogesterone in normal men and children with congenital hyperplasia. J Clin Invest 48:930, 1969
40. Lin TJ, Billiar RB, Little B: Metabolic clearance rate of progesterone in the menstrual cycle. J Clin Endocrinol Metab 35:879, 1972
41. Billiar RB, Jassani M, Saarikoski S, et al: Pregnenolone and pregnenolone sulfate metabolism in vivo and uterine extraction in midgestation. J Clin Endocrinol Metab 39:37, 1974
42. Tulchinsky D, Hobel CJ, Yeager EM: Plasma estrone, estradiol, estriol, progesterone and 17-hydroxyprogesterone in human pregnancy. Am J Obstet Gynecol 112:1095, 1972
43. Lin TJ, Lin SL, Erlenmeyer F, et al: Progesterone production rates during the third trimester of pregnancy in normal women, diabetic women and women with abnormal glucose tolerance. J Clin Endocrinol Metab 34:287, 1972
44. Billiar RB, Little B, Kline I, et al: The metabolic clearance rate, head and brain extractions and brain distribution and metabolism of progesterone in the anesthetized female monkey (Macaca mulatta). Brain Res 94:99, 1975
45. Baulieu EE, Godeau F, Schorderet M, et al: Steroid-induced meiotic division in Zenapus laevis oocytes: surface and calcium. Nature 275:593, 1978
46. Kopu HT, Hemminki SM, Torkkeli TK, et al: Hormonal control of uteroglobin secretion in rabbit uterus. Biochem J 180:491, 1979
47. Wambach G, Higgins JR: Antimineralocorticoid action of progesterone in the rat: correlation of the effect on electrolyte excretion and interaction with renal mineralocorticoid receptors. Endocrinology 102:1686, 1978
48. Landau RL, Bergenstal DM, Lugibihl K, et al: The metabolic effects of progesterone in man. J Clin Endocrinol Metab 15:1194, 1955
49. Castracane VD, Jordan VC: The effect of estrogen and progesterone on uterine prostaglandin biosynthesis in the ovariectomized rat. Biol Reprod 13:587, 1975
50. Rao CV: Inhibition of (^{3}H) prostaglandin F_2 binding to its receptors by progesterone. Steroids 27:831, 1976
51. Schwarz BE, Milewich L, Gant NF, et al: Progesterone-binding and metabolism in human fetal membranes. Ann NY Acad Sci 286:304, 1977

52. Csapo A: The four direct regulatory factors of myometrial function. p. 13. In Wolstenholme GE, Knight J (eds): Progesterone: Its Regulatory Effect on the Myometrium. Churchill, London, 1969

53. Fainstat T: Ureteral dilatation in pregnancy: a review. Obstet Gynecol Surv 18:845, 1963

54. Turkington RW, Hill RL: Lactose synthetase: progesterone inhibition of the induction of alphalactalbumin. Science 163:1458, 1969

55. Backstrom T, Baird DT, Bancroft J, et al: Endocrinological aspects of cyclical mood changes during the menstrual cycle or the premenstrual syndrome. J Psychosom Obstet Gynaecol 2:8, 1983

56. Garris DR, Billiar RB, Takaoka Y, et al: In situ estradiol and progestin (R 5020) localization in the vascularly separated and isolated hypothalamus of the rhesus monkey. Neuroendocrinology 32:202, 1981

57. MacLusky NH, McEwen BS: Progestin receptors in the rat brain: distribution and properties of cytoplasmic progestin-binding sites. Endocrinology 106:192, 1980

58. Bixo M, Backstrom T, Winblad B: Regional progesterone accumulation in the brain of the estrus rat. Acta Soc Med Suec 91:142, 1982

59. Batra S, Grundsell H, Sjoberg N-O: Estradiol-17β and progesterone concentrations in human endometrium during the menstrual cycle. Contraception 16:16, 1977

60. Merryman W, Boiman R, Barnes L, et al: Progesterone anesthesia: in human subjects: J Clin Endocrinol Metab 14:1567, 1954

61. Holzabauer M: Physiological aspects of steroids with anaesthetic properties: review article. Med Biol 54:227, 1976

62. Majewska MD, Harrison NL, Schwartz RD, et al: Steroid hormone metabolites are barbiturate-like modulators of the GABA receptor. Science 232:1004, 1986

63. Gyermek L, Genther G, Fleming N: Some effects of progesterone and related steroids on the central nervous system. Int J Neuropharmacol 6:191, 1967

64. Backstrom J, Langren S, Zetterlund B, et al: Effects of ovarian steroid hormones on brain excitability and their relation to epilepsy seizure variation during the menstrual cycle. In Porter RJ et al. (eds): Advances in Epileptology: XVth Epilepsy International Symposium. Raven Press, New York, 1984

65. Jouan P, Samperez S: In Motta M (ed): The Endocrine Function of the Brain. p. 95. Raven Press, New York, 1980

66. Holzbauer M, Youdim MBH: The oestrus cycle and monoamine oxidase activity. Br J Pharmacol 48:600, 1973

67. Ladisich W: Influence of progesterone on serotonin metabolism: a possible causal factor for mood changes. Psyconeuroendocrinology 2:257, 1977

68. Casper RF, Bhanot R, Wilkinson M: Prolonged elevation of hypothalamic opioid peptide activity in women taking oral contraceptives. J Clin Endocrinol Metab 58:582, 1984

69. Casper RF, Alapin-Rubillovitz S: Progestins increase endogenous opioid peptide activity in postmenopausal women. J Clin Endocrinol Metab 60:34, 1985

70. Sandberg AA, Slaunwhite WR Jr: The metabolic fate of C^{14}-progesterone in human subjects. J Clin Endocrinol Metab 18:253, 1958

71. Ottosson UB: Oral progesterone and estrogen/progestogen therapy. Acta Obstet Gynecol Scand [Suppl] 127:5, 1984

72. Smith SL, Cleghorn JM, Streiner DL, et al: A study of estrogens and progesterone in premenstrual depression: the family. p. 538. In: Tel Aviv, Israel: Fourth International Congress of Psychosomatic Obstetrics and Gynaecology, 1974

73. Harrison W, Sharpe S, Endicott J: Treatment of premenstrual symptoms: critical review and update. Gen Hosp Psychiatry 7:54, 1985
74. Sampson GA: Premenstrual syndrome: a double-blind controlled trial of progesterone and placebo. Br J Psychiatry 135:209, 1979
75. Moos RH: The development of a menstrual distress questionnaire. Psychosom Med 30:853, 1968
76. Halbreich U, Endicott J, Schacht S, et al: The diversity of premenstrual changes as reflected in the Premenstrual Assessment Form. Acta Psychiatr Scand 65:46, 1982
77. Keith G: A study of the premenstrual syndrome and progesterone/placebo therapy. PhD dissertation, Walden University, 1985
78. Van der Meer YG, Benedek-Jaszmann LJ, Van Loenen AC: Effect of high-dose progesterone on the pre-menstrual syndrome; a double-blind cross-over trial. J Psychosom Obstet Gynaecol 2:220, 1983
79. Maddocks S, Hahn P, Moller F, et al: A double-blind placebo-controlled trial of progesterone vaginal suppositories in the treatment of premenstrual syndrome. Am J Obstet Gynecol 154:573, 1986
80. Dennerstein L, Spencer-Gardner C, Gotts G: Progesterone and the premenstrual syndrome: a double blind crossover trial. Br Med J 290:1617, 1985
81. Lane G, Siddle NC, Ryder TA, et al: Clinical research. Br Med J 287:1241, 1983
82. Heckel GP: Endocrine allergy and the therapeutic use of pregnanediol. Am J Obstet Gynecol 66:1297, 1953
83. Mabray CR, Burditt ML, Martin TL, et al: Treatment of common gynecologic-endocrinologic symptoms by allergy management procedures. Obstet Gynecol 59:560, 1982
84. Lorber CA, Cassidy SB, Engel E: Is there an embryo-fetal exogenous sex steroid exposure syndrome (effesses)? Fertil Steril 31:21, 1979
85. Nora JJ, Hart Nora A, Wexler P: How teratogenic are the sex steroids? Comtemp Ob/Gyn February:39, 1983
86. Katz Z, Lancet M, Skornik J, et al: Teratogenicity of progestogens given during the first trimester of pregnancy. Obstet Gynecol 65:775, 1985
87. Check JH, Rankin A, Teichman M: The risk of fetal anomalies as a result of progesterone therapy during pregnancy. Fertil Steril 45:4, 1986
88. Hargrove JT, Maxson WS: Hypnotic effect of oral progesterone therapy. In preparation.

11

Premenstrual Syndrome as a Legal Defense

Elizabeth Holtzman

For too long women's health issues have been ignored, overlooked, or trivialized. This serious lapse in the medical community has had unfortunate consequences. One consequence has been a lack of research done on menstrual changes and symptoms. These symptoms deserve to be taken seriously and studied thoroughly, with the goal of providing relief to women who suffer from them.

The need for further research, however, is not to be confused with the issue of premenstrual syndrome (PMS) as a legal defense, which should not be taken seriously. This so-called defense rests on the absurd and baseless claim that some women become criminally insane and are driven to violent criminal behavior in connection with their menstrual cycle. For obvious reasons the PMS defense has no legal credibility and furthermore has ominous implications for the advancement of the status of women.

PMS AS A LEGAL DEFENSE:
THE SANTOS CASE

The country's legal debate on this subject was fueled by a case that came out of Brooklyn, People v. Santos in 1981.[1] Shirley Santos, a 24-year-old mother of six, was arrested in December 1981 for striking her 4-year-old child. In April 1982 defense counsel moved to dismiss the charges, claiming that Santos was suffering from "premenstrual syndrome" at the time of the assault. The motion was denied.

In November 1982 the defendant pleaded guilty to the charge of harrassment. In court she withdrew all defenses (including PMS) and specifically admitted responsibility for her actions. She was sentenced to a 1-year conditional discharge, requiring that she cooperate with the city welfare agency, undergo psychological evaluation, and continue the counseling she had begun voluntarily.

By admitting responsibility Santos explicitly rejected the PMS defense, as it is based on the concept of nonresponsibility. (Under the PMS defense a

137

woman can argue that because of her menstrual cycle she loses control over her actions, is unable to formulate any intent for her actions, or in some fashion is legally insane.)

By withdrawing all defenses and admitting responsibility Santos showed her claim for what it was—hollow and without merit. Furthermore, the defendant said in a television interview, "My nerves, they're not that bad that I'm going to get up because my period came down and hurt my kid." On top of that, it appeared that at the time she struck her child she already had her period, which probably obviates any claim of PMS, which means *premenstrual* syndrome. (The time course of premenstrual symptoms is variable. Symptoms generally cease with the onset of menses, but on some occasions women have reported symptoms persisting into the first or second day of their menstrual period.)

RESEARCH FINDS NO PMS

The novelty of the PMS defense inspired my office (District Attorney, Kings County) to do extensive research on the subject. Our search demonstrated that there exists no single, discrete, specific, or well-defined disabling medical condition that can be called PMS. We reviewed some 3,000 medical periodicals published since 1971 in English and a variety of foreign languages, including German, French, Spanish, Russian, and Chinese. We also consulted leading psychiatrists, endocrinologists, and gynecologists around the United States. We conducted this research in 1982 and 1983.

The scientific evidence shows that what is called premenstrual syndrome is actually a variety of symptoms (more correctly called premenstrual changes) that occur in various women in different ways or combinations. Furthermore, these changes are such that mood, appetite, sleep, energy level, and sexual desire may be either increased or decreased; such bipolarity of symptoms is not usually associated with a "syndrome." The symptoms that some women experience in connection with the onset of menses may also be experienced by people who are not premenstrual; bloatedness, anxiety, irritability, and depression are symptoms with a great many causes that occur in men as well as women.

PREMENSTRUAL SYMPTOMS DO NOT
AFFECT COGNITIVE ABILITY

Although more research is warranted, in my judgment, to learn how to provide relief for the symptoms felt by some women in connection with the menstrual cycle, it is a serious mistake to believe that these symptoms constitute a well-defined medical condition that "drives women crazy" once a month or relieves women from criminal responsibility. Although women with mental illness may get worse premenstrually, most normal, healthy women do not experience significant premenstrual changes in cognitive or mental function. Cognitive abilities do not diminish in connection with the menstrual cycle.[2,3] Scientific literature does not support the concept that, as a result of the menstrual cycle, otherwise normal women forget the difference between right and wrong.

PSYCHIATRIC ILLNESS AND PREMENSTRUAL CHANGES

The most recent edition of the American Psychiatric Association's nomenclature[4] does not cite PMS as a specific psychiatric illness. Late luteal phase dysphoric disorder (LLDD) is listed in the Appendix as a "proposed diagnostic category needing further study." In addition, Dr. Irving Nichols, Director of Practice Activities of the American College of Obstetrics and Gynecology stated, "I am unaware of any scientific evidence that supports the position that there is a relationship between premenstrual syndrome and criminal behavior."

There may be some connection between aggravation of a preexisting mentally deranged condition and the menstrual cycle; but in terms of normal people without any sign of mental illness, we were unable to find any scientific evidence suggesting that there is a connection between the menstrual cycle and psychosis, insanity, or crime.

PREMENSTRUAL SYMPTOMS DO NOT LEAD TO CRIME: A MATTER OF COMMON SENSE

Let us turn from science for a moment to human experience and common sense. Our experience throughout history and today tells us that women do not commit crimes on a monthly basis and women do not become insane and violent with cyclic regularity once a month. More than 90 percent of crimes are committed by men. What is their excuse, as they clearly are not suffering from premenstrual syndrome?

If premenstrual tension makes women mad and drives them to commit crime on a monthly basis, our prisons should be overflowing with female criminals. But they are not. The fact of the matter is that there is an infinitesimally small number of women in prisons and an infinitesimally small number of women as defendants in criminal cases.

THREE OTHER CASES OF PMS AS A LEGAL DEFENSE

Despite the immense publicity given to the PMS claim as a legal defense, there are only four cases that we are aware of in the world: two in England and two in the United States (including the Santos case).

In November 1981 two Englishwomen asserted PMS as a defense to criminal responsibility. In one case the defendant was originally charged with murder after killing her lover by running him over in a car. She pleaded guilty to manslaughter and was sentenced to a 12-month conditional discharge. A second woman, Sandy Smith, was accused of menacing a police officer with a knife. She too was convicted of the crime and put on probation for 3 years. In neither case was PMS used or accepted as a means of avoiding criminal responsibility. Neither woman was aquitted of all criminal charges; both were convicted. Although the judges in these cases may have accepted the claim of PMS to reduce or "mitigate" sentences, we have no way of knowing whether that happened. Indeed, judges have been known to give lenient sentences in cases where PMS was never an issue.

The only case in the United States, aside from Santos, occurred in Colorado. The issue was raised not in a criminal case but in a bankruptcy case, Lovato v. Irvin.[5] The facts of the case were as follows. Irvin attacked Lovato with a butcher's knife, causing serious injury, and Irvin pleaded guilty to attempted felony assault. In a separate suit Lovato was awarded monetary damages for these injuries. Irvin went to bankruptcy court trying to get this debt discharged, claiming that she was suffering from PMS at the time of the attack. After an extensive hearing that considered the scientific evidence on PMS, the court rejected the defense, stating that its acceptability as an explanation for criminal conduct had not yet been established medically or legally and that the expert testimony proved "a lack of any general acceptance of PMS in the psychiatric community as an explanation for inappropriate behavior."[6] Once again, this defense was found to be groundless and indefensible.

PMS DEFENSE FROM A LEGAL VIEWPOINT

From a legal point of view the fact that cognitive abilities do not diminish and that women do not lose the ability to distinguish between right and wrong in connection with the menstrual cycle is significant. In order to claim insanity in New York State, one of two conditions must hold true: (1) the person can no longer tell the difference between right and wrong; or (2) the person does not know the nature and consequences of his or her actions. There is no scientific evidence showing that there is a medical condition connected with the menstrual cycle that causes otherwise normal women to lose either of those capabilities.

Another way in which PMS could have legal consequences would be to claim that it causes diminished capacity in the criminal, i.e., that a woman suffering from PMS could not formulate the intention to commit the crime. Intent is generally a prerequisite for most violent crimes. It is difficult to argue that a person cannot formulate the requisite intent if that person does not lose cognitive abilities.

There are two other aspects with regard to the significance of a claim of PMS in the legal system. One has to do with determining guilt or innocence. In none of the known cases was responsibility for a criminal act excused on the basis of a claim of PMS.

The other concerns using PMS as a mitigating circumstance to be taken into account in sentencing. In England, in one case the woman did claim PMS (possibly along with other things), and the judge gave her a sentence of conditional discharge (similar to probation). However, I have seen judges give women similar sentences in Brooklyn even when they do not claim PMS. In one case the woman starved her child to death, and the judge gave her probation. There was no claim of PMS. It is difficult to say why a judge imposes a particular sentence, but I do not believe that judges in the English cases said that they were imposing a more lenient sentence because of PMS.

EVEN FOR WOMEN WITH ACUTE PREMENSTRUAL STRESS, PMS IS NOT A VALID LEGAL DEFENSE

Proponents of the existence of PMS and its use in court give the following rationale: If PMS exists, and if it exists in extreme form in some women, and if these few women commit crimes as a result, they should not be deprived of a legitimate defense just because it may cloud the horizon of increasing rights and responsibilities of women. PMS proponents claim that in some women violent conduct is cyclic and that it coincides with the onset of menses. Moreover, they claim, the violence is caused by the onset of menses. These afflicted women supposedly are symptom-free, placid, and calm at other times of the month, but premenstrually they undergo personality metamorphoses and cannot control their conduct. Those forwarding this argument fail to realize that a claim of inability to control one's conduct, with only one minor exception in the criminal law, is not a legal defense, at least not in New York State.

We do not in the law generally accept the notion that loss of control is an excuse for committing violent crimes. If a woman becomes so angry that she goes out and hits someone, it is not a valid legal excuse that she could not control her temper. She can still be prosecuted for that act. The only circumstance in which loss of control may have a legal significance as a defense may be in reducing the degree of homicide—from intentional homicide to manslaughter—because there is a legal concept of a crime committed in the heat of passion. Under those circumstances the *degree* of legal culpability might be minimized, but loss of control is not an excuse for criminal behavior and it is not a basis for avoiding criminal liability.

Even the claim of drunkenness as a means of diminishing capacity is not a claim that the threshold of restraint or the threshold of willingness to respond to provocation has been crossed but, rather, that the drunk person cannot formulate the required intent because his or her mind is so foggy from drink. The issue of loss of control may have medical consequences or medical significance, but it does not have legal significance, and that is an important distinction to bear in mind.

PMS IS NO EXCUSE FOR CRIMINAL BEHAVIOR

Defendants raise all kinds of claims. There was a homicide case in San Francisco in which the defendant claimed that because he ate some candy beforehand he had a condition brought about by the sugar in his body and therefore should not be found guilty. In fact, the jury acquitted him. Similar claims have been raised from time to time. Far be it for me in any way to inhibit the imagination, the very lively imagination, of defense counsel. However, we must address the question of scientific evidence. Research suggests that there is no specifically defined syndrome that affects all women or even a large group of women. There have been no controlled scientific experiments showing that the menstrual cycle is causally connected with women's criminality—none whatsoever. We should, of course, look at the effects, the consequences, the menstrual cycle has for women and find effective treatment for the well-known symptoms of anxiety, depression, or irritability. Nevertheless, those symptoms in and of themselves do not constitute excuses for criminal behavior.

PSM DEFENSE: A GRAVE THREAT TO WOMEN'S EQUALITY

There are other serious consequences of accepting PMS as a legal defense. The issue must be viewed not only in a scientific and legal context but also in the context of women's equality. Frankly, I think that the PMS legal defense is the old hocus-pocus about women in a new guise. Throughout history the idea that a woman's menses made her unclean, somehow tainted, and impaired her has been central to the discrimination that has persisted against women. The idea that women monthly can become violent, raging criminals is just a rephrasing of an old stereotype. It is one thing to focus on the medical phenomenon that affects some women; it is another to say that premenstrual symptoms separately or collectively drive women to commit criminal acts and create irresponsible, hysterical, unaccountable, nonhuman persons once a month.

PMS seems to be just another way to reduce the humanity of women. Common sense and extensive research show that women do not lose control of themselves premenstrually, nor do they pose the imminent threat to society implicit in claims about PMS.

Furthermore, if the idea gains credibility that once a month women lose the capacity to control themselves and become in essence insane and thus not accountable for their actions, women may be adversely affected in other ways. There would be severe consequences for women who seek to hold responsible positions in society. Who would ever trust a woman as president of the United States? After all, giving her control over "the button" could threaten the survival of the world! No doubt that example seems nonsensical to us, but I assure you many people believe it.

Imagine the consequences for employment decisions. If someone came to an employer and said that a female employee once a month may go out and stab somebody, the employer would have a difficult time justifying hiring her. In such cases the employer might even have a responsibility not to hire the female applicant in order to protect other employees.

We must be very careful about the language we use. By talking about PMS we might cause women to believe there is such a syndrome. Many American women might think that there *is* a condition of raging hormones which turns them into Dr. Jeckyl/Ms. Hyde.

We much also be aware of how the concept could create serious barriers to the equal treatment of women and furthermore be used directly against them. For example, accepting the notion that PMS is a factor could harm women in custody battles. It would thus be perfectly plausible for a mendacious husband to claim that his wife had PMS, which made her violent and crazy once a month, representing a threat to the children. It could also be used as a means of justifying violent assaults on women. A husband might claim that because his wife becomes mad and raging once a month he must use physical force in self-defense.

CONCLUSION

In absolutely no respect is PMS a valid legal defense for criminal behavior. It is important to remember that in no case has this defense been used successfully. I believe it will never be used successfully in the United States, nor should it be. Furthermore, the use of PMS as a legal defense can have far-reaching adverse consequences for women that have not been adequately examined. The premise of the PMS defense is that women are slaves to their hormones, which is simply a new verse added to a too-familiar, outdated song. It is time we began writing new songs.

REFERENCES

1. *People v. Santos*: No. 1K046229 (N.Y.C. Crim. Ct. Kings County 1981)
2. Golub S: The effect of premenstrual anxiety depression on cognitive function. J Pers Soc Psychol 34:103, 1983
3. Sommer B: How does menstruation affect cognitive competence and psychophysiological response? Women and Health 8:53, 1983
4. American Psychiatric Association: Diagnostic and Statistical Manual of Mental Disorders, Third Edition, Revised. American Psychiatric Association, Washington, DC, 1987
5. *Lovato v. Irving*: 31. Bankr. 251 (Bankr. N.D. Colo. 1983)
6. *Lovato v. Irving*: 31. Bankr. 257 (Bankr. N.D. Colo. 1983)

12

A Consumer Organization's Perspective

Virginia Cassara

As a result of the 4 years I spent seeking help for serious premenstrual symptoms, I concluded that there is no such thing as objectivity. We like to think that science is neutral, but in actuality "facts" depend on the questions asked, how they are posed in relation to other things, and what researchers expect to find. The closest we can come to objectivity is to be honest about our subjective point of view. Then others, aware of our perspective, can evaluate the information we present and decide what to accept or reject. My point of view is based on my experience as founder and Executive Director of PMS Action, as a social worker who has counseled more than 500 women with premenstrual syndrome (PMS), and, most important, as an informed medical consumer who had to go to great lengths (ending in England in 1979) to get help for PMS.

PMS ACTION

Founded in March 1980, PMS Action is a nonprofit organization whose mission is to educate laypersons and professionals about PMS. Our basic premise is that PMS is a biochemical disorder. We also believe that progesterone therapy ought to be a treatment option for American women. Prior to the existence of PMS Action, it was not.

Thus far, PMS Action has provided information to 90,000 laypersons and to 10,000 physicians and other health care professionals. For the first 3 years of our existence, we provided direct service (counseling) to more than 2,000 women, often with family members. The direct service program was an interim measure necessitated by the lack of recognition of PMS among laypersons and professionals and by the lack of effective treatment within the medical community. Today, thanks in large part to PMS Action's educational outreach, that situation has changed. PMS Action has been instrumental in the development of medical resources—familiar with and willing to treat PMS—in the local and national communities. We phased out of the counseling program and today maintain a list of physicians nationwide who treat women with PMS. In order to receive referrals from PMS Action, progesterone therapy—in dosages in accord with Dr. Katharina Dalton's protocol—must be a treatment *option*. For most physicians to whom we refer, it is an alternative provided only after many other treatments have proved to be ineffective.

Since 1982 PMS Action has conducted comprehensive training sessions in major cities across the country that thousands of health care professionals have attended. The expansion of our training program resulted in a major move for the organization from Wisconsin to Irvine, California in 1984.

MYTHS ABOUT PMS

Based on 20 years of living with PMS and on 5 years of professional involvement with it, I take exception to and want to qualify some prevailing myths about women with PMS.

The first myth: *Premenstrual symptoms result from negative conditioning about menstruation, femininity, and sexuality.* This misconception presupposes that a woman associates her symptoms with her menstrual cycle. Many women experience symptoms for years before they connect them to their cycles, as symptoms may begin as long as 2 weeks before menstruation or as soon as 2 days after its cessation. My own symptoms began during my teens, but I was 31 before I realized they were in any way associated with my cycle. Prior to that I simply thought I was a manic-depressive who had been cheated of her mania.

Not surprisingly, this myth rests on another generalization about women: We have so little of importance on which to focus our lives that our concentration focuses instead on thoughts of where we are in our menstrual cycle. Many of us have better things to do than to spend time noting "Today is day 6 of my cycle. Today is day 17, etc."—a menstrual mantra, of sorts, upon which most are not meditating.

The second myth: *PMS is a convenient excuse*—excuse for what I am not sure. The implication is that women with PMS are inherently neurotic hypochrondriacs who do not want to carry their share of the load. On the contrary, women have been carrying an incredible load—the burden of guilt. They have been cloaked in it, in part, by the dominance of the psychoanalytic tradition in American medicine and its concept of "wrongthink": Women who experience these symptoms do not accept their sexuality or femininity, are immature and lack coping skills to reiterate a few of the all too common explanations. Just 15 years ago, the same explanations were offered to explain spasmodic dysmenorrhea.

Women are not shirking responsibility. Most bend over backward to assume responsibility for their actions. Health care professionals would be more truly helping professionals if they realized that women seeking help for PMS rarely tell the whole truth and nothing but the truth. They hide some symptoms, couch others, and downplay all of them deliberately out of guilt.

The third myth: *PMS is not a serious disorder because it is self-limiting and because emotional symptoms are not serious symptoms.* Yes, PMS is self-limiting. The symptoms do go away each month—but they also return, month after month, wearing the woman down with time. As for the second point, how easy for those who do not experience depression to minimize it. When evaluating the seriousness of an illness, people—including medical professionals —respond differently when they can see or palpate the source of pain. Consequently, when concern is expressed about the potential side effects of a particular drug, the main fear is "Will it 'X' number of years from now prove to be carcinogenic?" I think of a segment of "The McNeil-Leherer Report" that focused on whether a potent, injectible progestogen should be approved by the Food and Drug Administration (FDA) as a contraceptive. A physician representing International Planned Parenthood, favoring its approval, said, "It has been used on millions, internationally, without serious side effects. The only side effects we have seen are weight gain and depression." Who says the depression the prestigious physician alludes to is not a serious side effect?

The fourth myth is of recent vintage, developed in response to the fact that women are no longer willing to suffer silently. We hear it often: *Women seeking help for PMS are looking for simple answers.* On the contrary, our dissatisfaction stems from the simple answers dispensed to us in the past: "If the oral contraceptive doesn't work, you need a psychiatrist." Or, "If symptoms persist after a hysterectomy, they're 'all in your head.' " In fact, these simple answers are the most frustrating and least effective measure for treating women with PMS. A more honest answer brings a more positive response, e.g., "Much more is not known than known about PMS." Or, "I don't know how to treat you, but I'm willing to work with you." We are not emotionally fragile beings who need protecting. We are capable of dealing with reality.

Myth number five: *Women who report PMS symptoms are setting the women's movement back.* Certainly, there are those who use the emerging public awareness of PMS to buoy their preexisting prejudices. However, sexism is no more rational than racism. Those who use the "new disease" PMS to judge women incapable of being pilots, paleontologists, or presidents would have said 5 years ago, "Women can't hold responsible jobs because of their 'raging hormones.' " Awareness of PMS sheds some light on the stereotypes that are the precursors of prejudice.

Note this passage from *An Essay on Women.*

> *She has two different sorts of mood. One day she is all smiles and happiness. . . . There is no better wife . . . nor prettier. Then, another day, there'll be no living with her. You can't get within sight, or come near her, or she flies into a rage and holds you at a distance like a bitch with pups, cantankerous and cross with all the world. . . . The sea is like that also. Often it lies calm and innocent and still. . . . Then it will go wild and turbulent. . . . This woman's disposition is just like the sea's . . . since the sea's temper also changes all the time.*

The words were written by Semonides, a Greek poet, during the sixth century BC. For thousands of years mankind has been making generalizations about womankind. Like the sea. Hysterical. Irritable. Moody. Unpredictable. Unreliable. Undependable. Inconsistent. Irrational. There are those who, based on observations of some women some of the time, say that that is the nature of women. It is not. The adjectives do describe, however, the nature of a woman with PMS. That PMS is in the limelight is a positive thing, not just for the woman with symptoms and those close to her whose lives are directly affected. It is a ray of hope for society. When PMS is recognized, researched, and treated, the stereotypes will diminish.

Finally, let us address *the myth of progesterone as placebo*. We do not know why progesterone apparently works for so many. Anecdotal evidence based on Dr. Katharina Dalton's work over the past 30 years in England and anecdotal evidence from more than 10,000 women on progesterone with whom PMS Action has contact contradicts the placebo theory. Progesterone is not a panacea. It does not work for all women with PMS, but it works for many. Certain factors suggest that its effectiveness is not merely as a placebo.

First, most women on progesterone get better results with time. Physicians prescribe conservatively, and it often takes several cycles to arrive at the correct dose level. Moreover, women must learn to use the medication consistently in order to get optimal results. Second, if progesterone were indistinguishable from placebo, why were prior testaments not equally successful? By the time progesterone is prescribed for a woman, she has usually tried many of the following treatments: oral contraceptives, diuretics, antiprostaglandins, vitamin B_6, progestogens, tranquilizers, antidepressants, and even hysterectomy. These facts lead to a third factor suggesting that progesterone's value is unlikely to be that of a placebo. The placebo effect presupposes faith, a naive acceptance that an omniscient, omnipotent physician has *the* answer. Because progesterone therapy is a therapy of last resort, by the time women get to progesterone the prevailing emotion is fear. The thought, "This is my last hope. What if it doesn't work either?" This attitude is not conducive to the placebo effect. Experience suggests that progesterone's effect is more than a placebo effect, but from the individual consumer's point of view I would be remiss if I did not ask, "Does it matter?"

WHAT IS THE ANSWER?

We do not expect simple answers. PMS probably has both genetic and psychological predisposing causes as well as environmental precipitating and sustaining causes (e.g., stress-related and dietary). However, the extent to which the etiology of PMS is biochemical is far greater than science has realized. "Psychogenic" is a convenient label for "under-researched."

Likewise, we cannot look at PMS as simply a medical or a scientific problem to the exclusion of a social and political one. When I started PMS Action 7 years ago, few in the United States had heard of PMS. Despite the fact that Dalton had been consistently publishing for 30 years—and progesterone had been available in the United States for 40 years—progesterone therapy was not a treatment option for American women. Today it is, and the impetus has come, in large part, from consumers who have responded to PMS Action's message: that women have to assume some responsibility for the fact that premenstrual and menstrual symptoms have not been a health care priority.

PMS Action has emphasized that it is critical to speak up about the extent and severity of our symptoms. Some simplistically say that PMS has not been recognized because physicians are men and men do not care about the health care needs of the other sex. Our message is that we must take mutual responsibility for our health care. The diagnosis of PMS depends on charting, and who charts? The individual woman. After this step a woman must exercise responsibility for choosing among a wide array of providers and treatments.

The concept of mutual responsibility for our health care should be liberating for physicians who, in the past, have been expected to have all the answers. The data are not in. The challenge to scientists, academicians, and health care professionals is to emphasize the importance of accumulating data and, in the interim, to treat patients compassionately and responsibly.

SUMMARY AND CONCLUSION

As a consumer and as founder and Executive Director of the national nonprofit organization PMS Action, the author addresses some prevailing myths about women with PMS. The assumption that negative attitudes about menstruation are responsible for premenstrual changes is challenged by the fact that many women do not associate their symptoms with their cycle. The assumption that PMS is a convenient excuse is challenged by the large number of working women with children and by the fact that dysmenorrhea was explained this way until the pathophysiology was understood.

The assumption that PMS is not a serious disorder is challenged by its chronic nature and severe mental pain. The suggestion that women are looking for simple answers is challenged by their willingness to work, stay in treatment, and change their life styles over a period of time. The fear that PMS is setting the women's movement back is challenged by a different perspective, i.e., not recognizing that PMS perpetuates stereotypes detrimental to women. Research is clearly needed, but in the interim women must assume a great deal of responsibility for their health care, and medical professionals have a responsibility to treat women with PMS.

ACKNOWLEDGMENTS

Work leading up to this chapter was sponsored by grants from the National Science Foundation and the National Endowment for the Humanities.

Index